Fibromyalgia Fatigue
and
You

Michael C. Kelly MRCPI
CONSULTANT RHEUMATOLOGIST

KELMED PUBLICATIONS LTD
IRELAND

PROFESSIONAL COMMENTS

Fibromyalgia is a major cause of impaired quality of life for many people. As the new millennium approaches, there is an emerging consensus as to both the physiological and psychological mechanisms which lead to pain amplification, fatigue, and somatic distress.

Dr Kelly has done patients a great service by writing this book, which is sympathetic to their plight and offers hard-headed practical advice. For some fibromyalgia patients, this book is all you will need. For other, acting on its advice will provide an ideal background for a meaningful collaboration with your doctor. Read this book not once but often and you will establish the groundwork for a more meaningful and less painful existence.

Overall I would rate this book as a courageous contribution, given the tendency to trivialise the fibromyalgia problem.

Robert M. Bennett, MD. The Oregon Health Sciences University, USA.

I find it interesting how much of what I tell my patients is written in this book. I think that it is an important message and that it should be communicated. There are not enough people out there saying the important things Dr Kelly is saying. This is an incisive and courageous appraisal of fibromyalgia and its treatments and an important book for all patients with fibromyalgia.

Frederick Wolfe, MD. Kansas University School of Medicine, USA.

I have read this book with considerable interest. I was very impressed by the comprehensive manner in which fibromyalgia is explained to the non-medical reader. This book outlines how this disorder has become increasingly understood in recent years but that there is still some way to go before fully understanding the pain and fatigue mechanisms involved. I think the book is realistic, practical and makes no unwarranted claims. For those who struggle under the burden of fibromyalgia, this book provides valuable insight and advice.

Professor Barry Bresnihan, Dept. Rheumatology, University College Dublin, Ireland.

This is a splendid book which will be very well received by patients. It explains in non-technical terms the background to this elusive malady, and gives a very balanced, sensitive and coherent approach to its management. I think this is a practical handbook that will be of great benefit. I particularly commend the sections on what can be helpful in treatment and also commend the important guide to what does not work. I certainly would be happy to recommend this book to my patients.

Professor Simon Wessely, Kings College Medical School London SE5 8AZ, England.

Prologue

The writer of this book heard very little of fibromyalgia during his student years and little more during early post-graduate training. However, he encountered many patients with this disorder at various rheumatology clinics. These patients usually consisted of a group of very dissatisfied sufferers who had many different diagnoses and who, as individuals, rarely responded to the multiplicity of treatment that was provided for them.

Many were regarded as having some form of depression or psychological abnormality.

Some had been previously diagnosed as having fibrositis but this diagnosis had fallen into disrepute at the time. In spite of the different diagnoses that all of these people had there was a sameness about them that suggested that they had a singular, if not easily identifiable, disorder and that they represented a specific sub-group of patients.

In the early 1970s articles began to appear in rheumatology journals, regarding people with 'fibrositis syndrome' or fibromyalgia.

The description of these patients and the difficulties in eradicating their symptoms mirrored the experience of this author.

So, now at least there was a diagnosis. While patients were pleased with this, treatment was still unsatisfactory and a cure remained elusive.

As treatment was so unsatisfactory the author produced various pamphlets to educate people with fibromyalgia about the nature of their condition and how they could help themselves. Many responded very well to these pamphlets and they were updated to the status of booklets, culminating in this latest effort. It is hoped that this will help victims of fibromyalgia to conquer the condition and so lead a life of normal health and vitality.

CONTENTS

Part One
Learning about fibromyalgia

1. Introduction 3
2. The diagnosis 9
3. What is fibromyalgia? 16
4. The symptoms of fibromyalgia. 25
5. Pain and exhaustion 33
6. Life with fibromyalgia 42
7. Standard investigations and treatments. 51
8. What causes fibromyalgia? 61
9. Other suggested causes of FM 67
10. Treatments available 82

Part Two
Revitalisation

11. Introduction 93
12. First steps 95
13. Physical fitness 101
14. Renewing friendships 104
15. Pain-relieving strategies 105
16. Fatigue-relieving strategies 110
17. Progress 111
18. The last lap. 114
19. The attitude of others towards you. 117
20. Your attitude towards others 124
21. Attitudes towards self. 126
22. Can anyone help? 129
23. Further progress 134
24. Life after fibromyalgia 137

Part One

Learning about fibromyalgia

Introduction

Fibromyalgia (FM) is a very common disorder.

It is not known what causes fibromyalgia even though there is alot of research taking place in many medical centres, particularly in the western world. Doctors disagree about its cause and indeed about its management. There is nothing at all surprising about this aspect of FM.

It afflicts people of all ages throughout the world. It is estimated that it afflicts over two per cent of the population in the United States. Some people consider that this figure may be an under-estimate, and that it may be even higher in some other countries. Regardless of the true figure it is an extremely common disorder. Its incidence in some parts of the world is not known, as it may well have a completely different name.

There is widespread acceptance among rheumatologists that it is the most common chronic painful condition they encounter in clinical practice. It is believed to be even more common than symptomatic osteoarthritis. Given that osteoarthritis is predominantly a disease of the elderly, it is clear that fibromyalgia is far and away the most common chronic painful condition in younger and middle aged people throughout the world.

However, there are a host of other interested bodies that are endeavouring to have their say, and for this reason FM has a high degree of controversy associated with it. These various parties, for their own reasons, want to belittle FM and relegate it to a medical nonsense.

In some countries where FM is regarded as a cause of disability, it is in the interests of insurance underwriters to degrade the condition and they frequently quote 'medical evidence' that suits their case, to achieve their aims.

Also included in these groups are some doctors who regard its many manifestations and the poor response to medication as evidence of its being at most a psychological disorder.

Even those who are sympathetic to people with FM have not helped the situation as they frequently insist that it is a very serious disease and use scant medical evidence to support their claims. Their wild claims are usually quickly discredited and this results in scoring opportunities for the opposition, which they seize upon with relief. Television debates on the topic do little more than entrench the views of the extremists on both sides.

Those occupying the middle ground continue to do the best they can for the fibromyalgia sufferers. While they continue to do that they are fully aware of the fact that medicine will not provide a cure of any sort, for a great number of years, if ever.

As contemporary medicine is not going to provide a cure, you may feel disappointed. This is understandable, even if it is somewhat defeatist on your part. However, having read this book you will not want anyone or any group of people to cure you as you will have developed a more enlightened perspective. You will want to overcome the condition largely by yourself.

Many authorities have suggested that you can help yourself but only in-so-far as they see fit for you. This book is different. It not only suggests that you should and indeed can help yourself, but it also suggests that, by your own efforts you can eradicate the scourge of FM completely.

At no stage is it suggested that this is going to be easy. On the contrary, it is a very difficult journey. However, success is attainable by your own efforts and the reward for success is that, not only will you beat the condition, but you will also learn much about yourself along the way. At the end of this journey you will enjoy a quality of life superior to what you enjoyed before fibromyalgia became such a major feature of your existence.

Part One of the book describes the symptoms of FM and the effects they have on the lives of sufferers. The physiological basis of the symptoms is also explained in a way that divests the condition of much of the ignorance in which it is shrouded. Lack of knowledge is one of the principal reasons for most people's inability to cope with the effects of the disorder.

Tangible explanations are put forward as to why you may have been susceptible to the development of the disorder in the first instance. With this knowledge you will also be in a position to understand why currently available treatments have so little to offer you. This will further encourage you to adopt the self-help route and will be a source of strength to you when the going gets rough.

Part Two of the book offers some general guide-lines that sufferers will find helpful on the road to recovery.

This book demands great effort on your part both in understanding the nature of the disorder and in implementing the life changes necessary to become well again.

It is not a lazy person's guide to success. It demands that you should have an open mind in spite of the fact that you may previously have absorbed much of the negative nonsense that is written about fibromyalgia. It demands the intellectual capacity to understand what is written and a persistent fortitude to then move on to normal health.

This book points you in the right direction. If you have the energy to move forward then at least you will be heading in the direction of normal health and vitality.

Many people who once were FM sufferers, who regarded themselves as chronically diseased patients and who were serious consumers of orthodox and alternative medical products have successfully overcome FM by the route suggested here. They are now ordinary healthy folk.

This might seem like an astonishing claim given the fact that so many of your previous efforts ended in failure, but nevertheless it is true. There is no reason at all why you should not also be successful.

Who gets fibromyalgia?

In this author's experience about 95 per cent of FM suffers are female though in other countries the female preponderance is not quite as high as this. No one knows why females should be more vulnerable than males, to this disorder.

There is certainly no hormonal, gynaecological or psychological reason for it. Women virtually never report that symptoms are more difficult to tolerate at the time of menstruation or indeed menopause.

This is somewhat surprising as certainly disorders such as migraine or back pain are very often described as being worse in the pre-menstrual phase.

FM affects all age groups from childhood upward. Likewise it afflicts people of all different cultural backgrounds, whether they reside in their native environment, or not.

This latter assertion is of vital importance as it clearly indicates that FM is not a modern disorder of western society as many would like to suggest.

Understanding fibromyalgia

Part One describe the symptoms of fibromyalgia and the effects they have on the lives of its sufferers. The information provided here is not taken from any texts or pamphlets on the condition. Rather it is information that has been directly gleaned from many hundreds of people with this disorder over a long period of time.

It is, in reality, a general account of the lives of many sufferers.

Other features that will be addressed here include the cause of the pain, the fatigue, the many other symptoms, and the links between them. Obviously, comments on these aspects rely on up-to-date medical research on what is known of the mechanisms of pain and pain control in human beings. They are also based on current understanding of the physiology of sleep.

Excellent research, carried out by many dedicated people over the years, provides this information and while this book advocates self-reliance, it never deigns to be disrespectful to, or in any way patronise the efforts of very many dedicated people who in their own way have helped many FM sufferers and who no doubt will continue to do so. Other factors such as the poor response to various medications will also be addressed.

In essence, I am making available to you the more practical aspects of recent research. Less emphasis is placed on research efforts that have not as yet translated into practical beneficial material.

The general thrust of this is strongly positive, and the scant regard in which naïve, useless or deliberately misguided treatments are held, should not to be interpreted otherwise.

It is one of the basic assumptions of this book that all victims have the inherent ability to understand the concepts explained here, and the desire and strength to get well.

To do this, your single most valuable asset is information. As in any conflict, and conflict this is, you must know and understand the enemy before it can be conquered.

The Diagnosis

Fibromyalgia is diagnosed on what doctors term clinical grounds. This means that its presence is confirmed on the basis of what you tell the doctor and on his or her finding tenderness in the areas of your body considered significant by the American College of Rheumatology (ACR). The diagnosis should be made by a properly qualified and competent doctor to rule out other disorders such as arthritis or degenerative changes in the spine that can give rise to somewhat similar symptoms.

Some other serious disorders can give rise to muscular pains but a doctor will be able to rule-out these on the basis of an examination with or without blood tests, or appropriate x-rays. Other disorders that can cause diagnostic confusion include Systemic Lupus, Erythematosis, Lyme disease, Polyarteritis Nodosa, some forms of Myositis and in the older age groups Polymyalgia Rheumatica.

The situation is further confused by the fact that some blood tests can give borderline results and therefore, clinical assessment of the patient is of critical importance.

Indeed it is accepted by many doctors and rheumatologists in the United States that people are wrongly diagnosed as having Lyme disease when in fact they have FM. This should help you appreciate the limitations of blood tests and the absolute importance of a proper medical assessment.

Many people with FM (as do others who have not got FM) have spondylitic spinal changes on x-rays. The contribution of these changes, if any, to the pain levels in every person with FM, needs to be accurately determined in order that appropriate treatment can be recommended. This further emphasises the importance of a proper medical examination.

The vast majority of people, because they read so many stories in the popular press about advances in medicine, believe that advanced technological tests get to the root of all disorders.

Indeed, many new medical graduates labour under the same false notions. The results of all tests have to be assessed in the context of the patient's symptoms and the findings on physical examination. Therefore, technological diagnostic advances are of little use, unless assessed by a sensible doctor. This is of particular significance in FM, as many people with fibromyalgia have a tremendous number of tests.

For instance scans nearly always reveal some abnormalities, especially in the spine, and if they are not properly interpreted, they can lead to a wrong diagnosis and the implementation of useless and sometimes dangerous treatments.

In today's world the benefits of a good family physician are very frequently overlooked. It is of vital importance not just in FM but in all medical conditions that you are assessed by a competent doctor.

You may feel that undue emphasis is placed on the role of your family doctor and that the above paragraphs are little more than a promoting of fellow professionals. It is the experience of this author that one of the most important drawbacks to people with FM making progress, is misinformation they have been given by alternative practitioners.

Another major disadvantage of tests is the fact that some people with FM insist that their symptoms must relate to some irrelevant abnormalities that were turned up in the course of investigations. Fibromyalgia is very easy to diagnose by any experienced clinician.

You will, in this book, read about the symptoms of fibromyalgia and how they affect you. By and large, from reading this, you will know if you do or do not have FM.

Fibromyalgia occurs in many people who have other disorders. People with arthritis or with mechanical back pain can and often do develop fibromyalgia. Such people believe, not surprisingly, that the added symptoms represent a deterioration in their original condition. Only your doctor can help determine the relative contributions of the original disease and the newly arrived FM to your current state.

Your doctor by doing so will ensure that you are getting appropriate treatment rather than increasing the treatments you were taking for the pre-existing arthritis, for instance.

While this book advocates self-reliance, you do need your doctor to determine your health status at the early onset of FM and perhaps later on at your discretion.

Misinformation about FM is one of your greatest enemies and there is a tremendous proliferation of this at the present time. Indeed if you accept the general thrust of this book, there should be no reason at all why you should not be able to raise any of the points made here with your doctor.

While medical tests, by and large, are of no great help except to rule-out other diseases, the same cannot be said of spurious tests that allegedly show that you are deficient in some vitamins or minerals or that you are allergic to every-day foods or substances that you come in contact with.

Many people with FM are delighted to get some diagnosis such as an allergy to something or other, or an infection of some sort or another.

It is human nature to wish to have a clear-cut black and white diagnosis with a clear-cut treatment rather than a complex disorder such as FM.

While it is human nature, it is also lazy. All such simplistic diagnoses achieve is ensuring you remain a patient and suppress your inherent ability to become well. Furthermore, many health foods and natural products are harmful.

They may not have been subjected to anything like the rigorous testing pharmaceutical products undergo before they are allowed on the market.

The American College of Rheumatology (ACR) has decreed that the presence of wide-spread pain and the presence of tenderness to touch in a given number of areas is sufficient to make a diagnosis of FM. However, many doctors are not fully happy with the criteria, but they remain as good as any other, to date.

All doctors who deal with people with fibromyalgia appreciate that there is much more to the disorder than mere pain alone.

The same of course applies to people who actually have the condition and who know perfectly well that it is not just a pain problem. In day-to-day practice, rigorous reliance on the presence of pain and tender points only, can lead to a failure to appreciate the full impact of fibromyalgia on the lives of sufferers.

You may well wonder why if the ACR criteria are not entirely satisfactory, that they are not altered to something more suitable. The reason for this is that there are many researchers in many countries throughout the world working on fibromyalgia. Such scientists in order to properly communicate and compare the results of their research, need to have strict criteria for diagnosis and response to treatment. The ACR criteria provide this and so avoid a Tower of Babel type situation where researchers in one country cannot understand and communicate with workers in other areas of the world. Therefore, the criteria while not perfect by any means, serves a very useful research function, though they may well be modified in future.

Pain is the major factor in the lives of most people with FM. As such, if referral to a specialist clinic is considered necessary for any reason, it is usually to a rheumatology clinic. Most of the researchers in fibromyalgia are rheumatologists and it is at rheumatology clinics that there is the greatest level of accumulated practical experience on the subject.

Indeed were it not for rheumatologists in Canada and the United States, fibromyalgia would still be conveniently regarded as a non-disease or a manifestation of some form of psychological inadequacy or even a manifestation of depression.

Likewise at these clinics there is some degree of understanding as to how the symptoms interact to make fibromyalgia such a miserable disorder. While you may not appreciate it, doctors are often very frustrated by the lack of efficacy of treatment in many of the serious diseases they deal with. This frustration is even greater when they try to help people with FM.

It is important that you should realise that fibromyalgia is not difficult to diagnose by doctors experienced in dealing with it, and important to also realise that you should not have endless tests carried out to see if "anything else" can be found.

If patients are not making progress they tend to have difficulty in understanding why this should be so. This is especially the case with FM, a condition most will have been advised is not serious, but is a condition which can impinge on life quality to an enormous extent.

So while a doctor may say to you that FM is not medically serious he or she will usually appreciate the serious effect it is having on your life.

After some time, doubts about the diagnosis may arise in the sufferer's mind. Even if these are not voiced, the doctor will be aware of them.

At any rate, these doubts may lead to your putting pressure on your doctor to do even more tests, the limitations of which have already been alluded to. These serve no useful purpose and they can also lead to a further delay in your accepting the diagnosis, making attempts to properly understand it, and embarking on the appropriate course of action.

A small number of medical practitioners have very little understanding of FM. These doctors will carry out numerous investigations in an attempt to come up with what they consider a real diagnosis. Only when they fail to do so will they reluctantly make a diagnosis of FM. This attitude betrays a lack of understanding of FM and also betrays the fact that the particular practitioner is unlikely to be helpful on your very difficult road ahead.

On the other hand some doctors will call any painful condition which they cannot understand, fibromyalgia. They also are not likely to help you on the road ahead.

Either of these groups of practitioners are not likely to be helpful to you. Basically their attitude does no more than add to the general confusion that surrounds fibromyalgia.

Doctor's experienced in dealing with people with FM will never make such a diagnosis as a matter of convenience. They will know that it is a very difficult disorder for a doctor to deal with. They will also understand that it is one of the most difficult of disorders for a patient to contend with.

Doctors who make a diagnosis of FM know that they are faced with a person and a disorder that will greatly challenge their skills and reserves of energy. They also know that at the end of the day they may gain no more than the contempt of the patient, regardless of their efforts.

Nevertheless, it is true that many people who do not have FM have acquired just such a diagnosis. This fact has led to much further confusion and many unnecessary arguments between various specialists and indeed various vested interests, much to the disadvantage of people who really have FM.

What is Fibromyalgia?

Fibromyalgia (FM) is a very common disorder and is also a very unique one.

Its main features are widespread pain and tenderness. The most common areas of the body that are painful are those about the shoulders, extending towards the neck and the lower back towards what people know as their hip bones.

The front of the chest and some areas of the limbs are also frequently involved but overall the pain predominantly resides in the trunk or torso rather than the limbs. Some people with fibromyalgia will report that they have pain nearly everywhere.

The pains are felt in fleshy muscular areas of the body and at bony points, as opposed to arthritic pains which are located clearly and specifically in the joints. Fibromyalgia pain is usually well removed from joints.

Even when it is close by, its true location can be readily determined by a detailed physical examination carried out by a medical practitioner.

While pain is the major problem for most people, it is a feature that rarely occurs in isolation. It is usually accompanied by a wide variety of other symptoms. By symptoms are meant discomforts that people suffer that should not normally be present. The most important of these non-painful symptoms is fatigue.

For many sufferers pain is the dominant feature, but in others fatigue presents the greater burden. Varying combinations of both are present in all sufferers and together they represent a formidable burden and obstruction to living a life of normal quality.

Psychological distress, often manifested as mood changes and irritability, while not an integral part of the disorder, is frequently present. In a similar manner depression can become a feature of the disorder.

There are a variety of other problems that are encountered in the fibromyalgia population, in a higher incidence level than would be expected. Perhaps the most common of these is discomfort, or pain often accompanied by a feeling of swelling of the abdomen. An extraordinary number of people with FM have these abdominal symptoms and frequently they will have been diagnosed as having irritable bowel syndrome or spastic colon. Discomfort passing urine, sometimes referred to as recurrent cystitis or as irritable urethral syndrome, is fairly frequent.

Less common symptoms include intolerance to cold, heat, or noise and areas of pins and needles or numbness in the limbs.

Some people will complain of swellings of the fingers with tightness of rings, while others feel that their ability to concentrate or calculate is impaired, as indeed may be their memory. These secondary symptoms, while bothersome in their own right, are generally less of a problem than are the primary features of pain and fatigue.

In strict medical terms the defining features of FM are widespread pain and tenderness persisting over a period of some months at least. Many doctors who are familiar with fibromyalgia and its effect on its victims, are not entirely happy with this strict definition because of the frequent presence of many of the secondary symptoms listed above. Because of this they feel that the condition would be better named Fibromyalgia

Syndrome (FMS). A syndrome may be defined as the presence of a characteristic set of symptoms that points to the existence of a particular disorder.

In essence, there is much more to FM than pain. One can therefore appreciate and empathise with the views of many doctors who know that it is much more than a mere painful disorder. However, this book is not about semantics but rather your regaining health and vitality.

There is one other highly significant feature of fibromyalgia that is either overlooked entirely, or never receives the emphasis it deserves in any of the numerous publications on the subject to date. This feature is the poor response of the symptoms of FM to all of the treatments that are available, whether these treatments have some scientific rationale or whether they are of the alternative variety.

Indeed, it can be stated that if a patient can say that a particular line of medical or other treatment has resulted in a dramatic improvement, it makes the initial diagnosis of fibromyalgia very suspect. This poor response to treatment is one of the most frustrating and demoralising aspects of FM.

Unique features of fibromyalgia

Fibromyalgia has quite a unique position among all of the painful conditions that affect humanity. There are a number of reasons why this should be so. One of the most important is that the cause of the pain is so poorly understood. In today's world people expect medicine to provide adequate explanations for the cause of most symptoms, and indeed in many diseases, modern medicine does not disappoint.

The cause of pain in such diverse disorders as cancer, migraine, arthritis, and various infectious and inflammatory disorders is known. However, the cause of pain in FM is not clearly known. It is obvious to any doctor who talks to people with FM that this very fact is a source of considerable frustration.

The same lack of knowledge applies to the cause of the fatigue and to the cause of the many other symptoms that are present. The multiplicity of symptoms and how they combine to make life so miserable is yet another feature that is pretty unique to FM.

Patients with back pain due to a prolapsed disc, or joint pain due to arthritis, will have pain to deal with. They will have a logical explanation for their pain, at least if they attend a competent medical practitioner.

To understand the nature of one's symptoms helps all patients cope with their discomforts and disorders.

The person with FM has great trouble in coping with the manifestations of the disorder as no one can truthfully explain their causes in an adequate and easy to understand manner.

The pain of many diseases can be eased by the patient taking appropriate action to avoid aggravating the pain or by using medication. The pain of FM is uniquely resistant to the efforts of sufferers to help themselves and is equally resistant to the many medications that are availed of.

People with FM are usually continuously fatigued. The apparently logical answer to this is to do less, and to sleep more. Yet, no matter how much the victims of FM sleep or rest, they remain as fatigued as ever.

In essence the variety of symptoms, the manner in which they combine to make life so miserable, the difficulty in understanding their causes, and the frustrating inability of treatments to significantly modify them, bestows on fibromyalgia a unique place among the many medical disorders encountered.

You may note at this stage that the term disease has been used in the text in some instances but it has not been applied to FM, for reasons that will later be discussed.

As the cause of the pain in FM is so poorly understood and as current-day medications offer such poor respite, you may feel that there is little to be gained in reading further. However, the emphasis here is positive, and indeed, very positive.

This book advocates self-reliance rather than a one-dimensional expectation that somehow medical science should shake itself up and provide for you an external solution to a disorder that is very often totally controlling your life.

The situation is far from hopeless and the excellent research that has been done over the last thirty years, whilst not cracking the problem, has thrown fresh light on the physiological mechanisms of pain, fatigue, and indeed many other symptoms of fibromyalgia.

The appreciation of the nature and cause of the symptoms, and how they affect people, is improving. The medical understanding of the mechanisms of pain and pain control, is likewise improving. This provides hope for better medicines in the distant future and also provides for sufferers an understanding of the basic concepts that will enable them to first understand, then come to terms with, and finally liberate themselves from one of the most miserable medical conditions of all.

Is fibromyalgia new?

The term fibromyalgia is a relatively new addition to medical dictionaries. The condition itself is far from new. It has been described in medical texts as far back as medieval times though under many different names.

In 1904 "fibrositis" was described in the *British Medical Journal* in an article written on lumbago. A word ending with "itis" implies inflammation. Tonsillitis means inflammation of the tonsils just as sinusitis means inflammation of the sinuses.

It was initially thought that there was inflammation in tissue fibres at the sites of low back pain, hence the term "fibrositis". It was then, as it is now, a very difficult condition both for the patients and indeed the doctors whose role it was to cure all ailments.

Over the years many doctors felt uncomfortable with fibrositis since it did not respond to treatment as did other diseases. In a sense it challenged their sense of infallibility and undermined their usual sense of being in control. In the 1950s and 1960s with the advent of new anti-biotics and other new treatments for many diseases, the medical world was full of enthusiasm. All diseases were tackled with a brave new confidence. However, in the fibrositis world nothing changed. This increased the levels of frustration felt by many doctors.

For some, frustration turned to doubts about the physical authenticity of the disorder.

The next stage in the evolution of the attitudes of some doctors was scepticism. The obvious psychological distress of some patients with fibrositis provided further ammunition for some sceptics who wished to have the entity relegated to a non-disease or to something that was 'all in the head'. From a medical point of view that was the lazy way out.

Advances in microscopy led to the discovery that there was none of the postulated inflammation in the painful tissues. This was all the critics needed to discredit the entity entirely.

Out of this was born a generation of doctors who feared to speak of fibrositis lest they be considered fringe practitioners. Publishing a paper on the subject, other than belittling it, would not have been a wise career move for any doctor who wished to make any progress in academic medicine.

All through this time people with FM were neglected by the medical profession. They often went elsewhere and picked up diagnoses such as 'Candidiasis', 'Myalgic encephalomyelitis' and of course allergies to all and sundry. In reality the absence of inflammation in the painful areas did nothing more than prove that the term fibrositis was a bad choice of title, chosen some sixty years beforehand.

Doctors who could appreciate that not all disorders of the human condition could be ruled in or ruled out, on the basis of tests, were silenced. Indeed, their confidence in dealing with such patients was undermined. This was a great disservice to fibrositis patients and the condition was almost apologetically referred to in medical texts if at all. It was treated as an embarrassing footnote, a legacy of less enlightened times.

However, highly motivated doctors refused to be cowered by the new orthodoxy, and continued to try to better understand the disorder.

As a result of their efforts in the early 1970s new criteria were laid down for the clinical diagnosis of the condition, using the new term 'fibromyalgia'. These were the antecedents of the most recent American College of Rheumatology criteria.

This research work resulted in a much greater understanding of the nature of the condition and the physiological basis of the symptoms encountered, which is of practical significance to all doctors and all people with FM. It is of particular significance to you on the road ahead, as knowledge will prove to be your greatest ally.

Is fibromyalgia becoming more common?

It is not possible to say if fibromyalgia is increasing in prevalence or not. It certainly is being recognised more than it was in the past. Likewise because of its new-found credibility doctors are not now afraid to make a diagnosis of FM. Therefore there are many more people now with a diagnosis of FM than there were a number of years ago. This is not really the same as to say that it is more common. In countries where FM is recognised as a cause of disability, it is the experience of insurance underwriters that payments for FM have increased alot over the past number of years. There is no doubt that in these countries, a large number of people are jumping on the FM band-wagon.

This is not only the opinion of this author but has been clearly stated by some of the leading doctors in America and Canada who themselves are very sympathetic to the FM construct and to the genuine sufferers of fibromyalgia.

This author practises in an environment where FM is not widely recognised or accepted as a cause of disability. In essence, he has gleaned his experience from a fibromyalgia population that has no conceivable secondary gain in having a diagnosis of FM and whose only desire is to be well again. This population of patients have not read of the symptoms of FM in some glossy magazine directed mainly at women. So there is no question of peer copying or adopting symptoms in order to assume the sick-patient role.

The incidence of FM has, in some countries, become a political, social and economic issue; this certainly applies to Canada, the United States and Great Britain. In the latter area people with FM have the label Myalgic Encephalitis (ME) which leaves the status of victims very vulnerable to genuine or vested interest group sceptics.

It is clear there are groups of people who want the condition again relegated to the status of a non-disease or a malingerers' charter.

This book does not concern itself with the interests of any *vested interest group* on any side of the arguments on any aspect of FM.

The true incidence of genuine FM is probably not much greater than it was years ago, but socio-economic and political influences may well have distorted the apparent incidence in some countries. The politics of FM are not within the brief of this book.

Neither is the question of disability in FM or whether anyone with fibromyalgia should or should not be considered fit for work which is also a very emotive and controversial topic.

This book aims to provide you with the means to move forward to normal health, so references to work incapacity are beyond its scope and should be of no interest to you as your sole ambition must be to regain normal health.

The Symptoms of Fibromyalgia

Pain is the over-riding factor in the day-to-day life of people with fibromyalgia. The pain of FM, while always to the fore, often varies in intensity from time to time. Bad spells are interspersed with periods when the pain is not quite so bad. Pain, however, is an almost constant companion. Well-conducted studies published in quality medical journals have revealed that people with FM suffer more from pain than do patients with rheumatoid arthritis, for instance. This is not the same as saying they have more severe pain. Such a statement surprises many observers who are not familiar with the syndrome, and who are not familiar with the gross inadequacies of the simplistic tests used to assess pain levels.

On face value, it does seem rather astonishing that people with FM who on physical examination are found to have little wrong medically, should report worse pain than patients with rheumatoid arthritis who on examination have swollen, inflamed, and sometimes deformed joints. Reasons for this apparent discrepancy will be dealt with later.

The basis of the pain of fibromyalgia differs from that of pain in conditions such as arthritis. Many FM sufferers have great difficulty in finding words to accurately describe their pain. Some will describe a constant aching, others will relate that they feel as if they were beaten up or run over by a car, while others have trouble in describing the pain as anything other than excruciating. The painful areas of the body are very tender to touch.

This is easy to detect on physical examination. Occasionally the tenderness is exquisite to the extent that even a shoulder strap may be uncomfortable.

On examination, people with such a degree of tenderness will frequently wince or withdraw from the touch in a dramatic fashion. A doctor without experience in FM may consider the situation unreal. He or she may then come to the conclusion that the person is either malingering or else has a psychological aberration as the cause of the problem. The person with FM often detects these doubts and this in turn leads to even greater difficulty in coping with the problem.

For many people pain is constant. A minority are more fortunate in that they may have reasonable periods of time without much pain. They often have painful periods interspersed with pain-free periods for some months. Indeed, some older patients, when the matter is probed more deeply, will relate that they had been diagnosed as having fibrositis many years previously, so clearly they have had some years without pain.

One way or the other, the presence of almost constant pain, the poor response to medication in the absence of a logical explanation, and the doubts of helpers all have a very frustrating and demoralising effect on people with fibromyalgia. Confusion, frustration and bewilderment render the pain experience of FM different and more difficult to cope with than the pain experience of a patient with arthritis. A distinction between severity of pain generally and the severity of any individual pain experience, is strongly emphasised in this book.

Those specialists who do not, who can not, or who will not accept that FM is a discrete, clear-cut, easily identifiable syndrome, argue that pain is a fact of life and that people with FM differ only in that they have a little more pain than average. They also argue that such patients have no other identifying features except that they are always conscious of it and always struggling to be 'cured' of what is essentially a normal state.

However, the pain quality, its intensity, its resistance to all medicines, and the widespread tenderness, strongly overcome any such arguments as does the striking similarity of these findings in nearly all people with fibromyalgia. Similar arguments about the cause and the nature of the fatigue, also, do not stand up to critical analysis.

Pain in both humans and animals is an unpleasant sensation but never-the-less one that is essential for survival. In animals, insofar as a human can understand, pain is merely one of the senses necessary for self-preservation. It serves as a warning to take appropriate action which usually means eradicating or escaping from whatever is causing the irritation or threatening survival.

In humans, with ongoing seemingly never-ending pain, it is an experience in suffering. The human can be frightened, bewildered, angry, confused, distressed and demoralised by pain and this certainly applies to the situation in fibromyalgia.

The pain sensation of a toothache or a broken arm can be very intense. However, such a pain, because it can be understood and eased to a certain extent by medication, can be coped with.

A much less intense pain from the chest or abdomen, which is not understood, can frighten the victim. In this situation, the pain, though not intense, is a bad experience. The ability to cope is diminished and the distress is all the greater. Clearly in humans there is much more to the pain experience than the actual intensity of the pain itself.

It is important to be aware of the difference between pain intensity, which may be the same for different people with similar conditions, and the pain experience which is unique to each individual and which is influenced by so many factors other than the severity of the pain.

In order to help you appreciate this point I will refer to the pain that is endured by people who have arthritis, for instance. The pain of this disease serves no purpose other than to inflict suffering. However, there is some understanding of the pain of arthritis. People with arthritis know why they have pain and so also do those who care for them whether it be family, friends, or medical personnel.

Sufferers are helped to cope and lessen the misery of the pain experience. Understanding the nature and cause of pain and indeed having family and friends who understand the situation, helps anyone with chronic pain to cope with it. Medications also help to a certain extent by lessening the intensity of the pain of arthritis.

Contrast this with the situation of the sufferer of fibromyalgia. Here the cause of the pain is not understood by the person who has the pain nor by those who would be helpful if that person had a disease that was readily understood.

In FM there is no inherent internal or external back up. You are on your own, isolated in your suffering and misery. Neither you nor others understand, and therefore your ability to cope is very logically at a low ebb. The pain experience of FM is one of lonely isolation and perpetual miserable suffering. This perhaps is the reason why people with FM place themselves so much higher on pain scales compared with people who, to casual observers, clearly have great pain.

The pain scale that is most commonly used is what is known as the visual analogue scale (VAS). This scale consists of a straight line with a zero marking at its left extremity, and a 10 rating at its right extremity. A person with pain is asked to mark her pain level on the scale. A mark at zero indicates no pain at all while a mark at 10 indicates the worst possible pain.

The person with little pain will put her mark close to zero while the patient with severe pain will put a mark closer to 10. This scale is used by doctors to assess the severity or intensity of the pain.

However, I believe that this method of testing makes no allowance for either the human factor or the human condition. While the doctor sees the mark as a level of the intensity of the pain, the patient is indicating the level of the misery of her pain experience.

As the pain experience of FM is such a devastating one, for a multiplicity of reasons, it is no wonder that the individuals with fibromyalgia mark themselves so high up on the scale.

These assertions, if correct, serve to demonstrate the fallibility of visual analogue scales, especially in people with FM. When used to compare pain levels of people with arthritis and the pain levels of people with FM, the test is not comparing like with like. In the patient with arthritis it may well give some indication of the intensity of the pain but in the person with FM it is, more truly, an index of the misery of her pain experience. At this stage you can now appreciate the difference between pain severity and severity of the pain experience. It is vital that both you and, more especially, those who care for you should understand and fully appreciate this difference.

This statement is not intended to demoralise you or to cause you to feel sorry for yourself. It helps you and those who wish to help you to understand the way you feel and what you have to confront. It should not engender self-pity but rather strengthen your resolve to become well again.

This is why at the beginning of this chapter it was stated that people with FM suffer more from pain though they do not necessarily have more pain than people with arthritis.

Fatigue in FM

Fatigue is present in virtually all FM sufferers. For some, pain is the most debilitating feature, while for others fatigue is more dominant.

Quite often pain and fatigue are equally troublesome and the combination greatly interferes with normal vitality and life quality.

If pain is the main feature the patient may be referred to a rheumatology clinic. If fatigue is the main problem the patient may be referred to a general medical department. There, after appropriate though sometimes over extensive investigations, a diagnosis of Chronic Fatigue Syndrome (CFS) may be made. Unfortunately in some cases a diagnosis of a psychological or psychiatric disorder is directly or indirectly implied.

In this author's opinion, FMS and CFS represent slightly different manifestations of the same underlying disorder. They are at the opposite ends of the same spectrum but a mix of both is the usual order of things.

The majority of people with predominant fatigue are labelled CFS. Some, unfortunately, get a diagnosis of post-viral-fatigue. This is unfortunate as it suggests you have a disease that needs a specific medical treatment. Regardless of what label you have procured, the same essential physiological mechanisms are giving rise to your problems. The road of recovery is also the same. This book asserts to be equally useful to you whether you have been labelled FM, or CFS.

Just as the pain of fibromyalgia has unique qualities, so also has the fatigue, and they are equally unpleasant. A farmer at the end of a day's work in the field may well feel tired.

This tiredness is natural and not at all unpleasant. It can be favourably modified and eased by any of many methods, rest, recreation or relaxation. Such healthy tiredness also invites healthy sleep.

Much more importantly such fatigue is eliminated by sleep.

This wholesome and healthy normal tiredness contrasts in many ways with the fatigue of FM. The fatigue of FM is an unnatural washed-out feeling. It does not resemble normal tiredness in any way. It is not eased by relaxation nor is it abolished by sleep.

People wake up exhausted in the morning. Even when they have slept for a normal period of time they feel as if they have not slept at all.

They are suffering from non-restorative sleep. This exhausted washed-out feeling of FM is present regardless of levels of activity and regardless of the amount of time spent sleeping.

Everyone is susceptible to fatigue and there is much discussion about the fatigue element of FM. Those who oppose the concept of FM as a distinct entity suggest that all people have varying degrees of fatigue, just as all people have varying levels of blood pressure. They argue that people with FM have a little more pain than average, and that they likewise have just a little bit more tiredness than normal.

However, it is not as simple as this. If it were, then extra sleep would lessen fatigue just as blood pressure pills might bring down blood pressure.

Also the exhaustion of fibromyalgia is a totally different experience to being a little more tired than average. It can readily be identified as such both by the victims themselves and by anyone who listens to what these sufferers are saying, especially if the listener has the ability to appreciate what is being said.

Psychological distress

Psychological distress, often manifested by mood changes such as irritability, tearfulness, and general frustration are present in people with FM. This is not surprising.

While not an inherent part of the condition, FM certainly brings its own problems and compounds the difficulties posed by the primary factors of pain and fatigue. Many will be disappointed that psychological distress is mentioned as they may already have had an excess of psychological explanations for their symptoms. Nevertheless it can become an important factor. This is not an *á la carte* production and if you are going to make progress you will have to consume all of its parts, even those you find not so much to your liking.

The irritability and mood changes frequently lead to people withdrawing from normal social activities. As a result, sufferers can lose their friends and further increases the misery of the disorder. Many with FM end up cocooned in a state of perpetual misery and isolation.

Depression

Depression can also be a major problem for people with FM. Depression broadly speaking can be divided into two types. The less serious type is a reactive depression that can occur in response to the misery of FM just like the psychological distress just alluded to. The second and more serious type is what is known as endogenous depression which can occur in any person with or without fibromyalgia. It is absolutely essential a medical assessment is made to determine if this latter type is present, as medical treatment may be required. The author is not suggesting that it is an inherent part of the syndrome, but if present in any individual, it must be assessed and treated appropriately.

Pain and Exhaustion

Pain is an unpleasant sensation caused by some injury to the body. It serves a very important function. For instance if a person places a finger on something hot he immediately feels pain which warns him to withdraw his hand before it is damaged.

Pain is a normal protective sensation. If it were not for the protection which pain sensitivity provides, serious damage would be incurred in day-to-day living.

If a person suffers nerve damage to his hand that leads to a loss of pain sensation, then that limb will be severely damaged unless well protected. Leprosy is a dramatic example of this. Pain, though unpleasant, is vital to survival.

Pain threshold

The appreciation of pain intensity must be confined within fairly strict limits. On the one hand the body must be able to interpret what may be injurious in order that appropriate action can be taken. On the other hand it must not interpret as injurious, normal day-to-day activities such as physical work, or the shaking of hands with a friend, or the pressure of clothes on the skin.

Low intensity stimulation does not register as discomfort until it exceeds what is known as the pain threshold for that given person.

Pain threshold varies between individuals. Some people have a low pain threshold. For these people it takes little to register as pain while the opposite holds for a person with a high pain threshold.

Everyone can appreciate that different people vary in their sensitivity to pain. However, it is not widely appreciated that any given person's pain threshold can vary from time to time.

An awareness of these points is absolutely fundamental to acquiring an understanding of what the pain of fibromyalgia is all about.

Pain threshold control

Pain threshold is normally constrained within very narrow confines. Any sensation that is detected by the skin or other tissues, for instance, is transmitted to the brain where it is interpreted as bad or not; appropriate action is then ordered by even higher brain levels.

All messages reaching the brain are influenced on their journey through the spinal cord and lower part of the brain by chemical mediators. Some of these facilitate the transmission of pain. Some of them do the exact opposite and actually dampen down the intensity of the pain message. There are many such chemical mediators. Perhaps the two that are most written about now are, serotonin, and substance P, but you will soon be reading of others.

There is a fine balance between pain-enhancing and pain-suppressing chemicals and this maintains the normal pain threshold. The balance can vary from time to time. If the balance is in favour of pain suppressors then the pain threshold is high and during such periods the person is relatively resistant to pain. If the balance favours the chemicals that augment painful stimulations, then it will take very little to register as pain. In such a case, the pain threshold is low in that individual.

In essence during these periods the person is very sensitive to pain. Thus, depending on the relative amounts of pain enhancers and pain suppressors in the brain and spinal cord, the pain threshold in any individual is variable.

People are actually aware of this in practical terms. For instance, a footballer who is warmed up in the heat of a game can take tackles from which he will feel no pain, until perhaps he cools down. Basically this is because during intense physical activity the brain is pumping out pain suppressors or natural pain-killers, so the pain threshold is very high.

At the other end of the scale we are all aware of the fact that if we are very tired or perhaps suffering from flu, it will take very little knocking about to cause alot of pain and discomfort.

This is because chemicals that heighten pain awareness are in the ascendancy and the pain threshold is low.

These natural alternations in pain threshold must be understood by all people with FM as part of building their solid foundation of knowledge, from which progress can be made.

Relevance to fibromyalgia

In arthritis, pain is caused in most cases by inflammation of the lining of the joint which is red and angry and which is producing chemicals that irritate nerve endings and send strong pain signals to the brain.

In other words there is a disease process in the joints that logically gives rise to pain.

We have already alluded to the fact that there is no inflammation in the tissues that are painful and tender in fibromyalgia. In fact, there is very little evidence that there is any abnormality at all in the painful areas though some poorly conducted trials have suggested as much. Certainly there is no abnormality in muscles that might even remotely give rise to the degrees of pain experienced by people with FM.

How then can pain be explained in these areas? Many experts believe that the pain in fibromyalgia has nothing at all to do with any disease in the painful areas and everything to do with the control of pain threshold. (By experts I mean people who despite the limitations of knowledge, carry out genuine research for the benefit of fibromyalgia victims rather then people of self-professed expertise who wish to sell products to a vulnerable group of people.)

More accurately it is thought to be due to a breakdown in the normal pain control mechanisms leading to a lowering of the pain threshold. It is felt that the pain is due either to an excess of pain enhancers or else a deficiency in pain suppressors, or a combination of both. In any case, the balance is upset and it now favours pain facilitation or easy expression of pain.

The overall effect is one of greatly lowering the pain threshold.

When the pain threshold is a little lowered it results in tenderness and soreness to light touch, that normally would not give rise to pain. When it is lowered still further a number of areas of the body register as being painful all of the time even when there is no pressure on them. This occurs without the necessity for the presence of any disease in the painful areas. There is no disease in the painful areas: only the presence of pain.

You can now appreciate the basis of the earlier assertion that the pain of fibromyalgia has an entirely different basis to that of any other condition.

If a tooth is painful there is something wrong with the tooth; if a joint is painful as in arthritis there is something wrong with the joint; but yet when some part of the body is painful in fibromyalgia, there is strikingly no disease in the painful area.

It is this totally different origin of pain that bestows on fibromyalgia pain many of its unique characteristics. It goes a long way towards explaining why the pain is so resistant to medications that in other conditions provide such good, if not total, pain relief. It also goes some way towards explaining why people with fibromyalgia have so much difficulty in describing the pain, understanding it and coping with it.

When you understand all of this, you are some way towards understanding what fibromyalgia is all about. You have also taken some steps on the road to success. At this stage you should know enough to be able to handle the assertion that pain in FM is not caused by any disease that doctors understand as a disease.

Fibromyalgia is a disorder, not a disease. Attempts at finding evidence for it being a disease and attempts at treating it as a disease at least in terms of 'the clinical model' are doomed to failure. In this book it is recognised as a disorder correctable by your own efforts rather than a disease which other people must cure you of.

Other implications

In fibromyalgia the pain threshold is lowered and non-diseased areas of the body are interpreted as being the source of the severe pain. That is the essential feature of the syndrome.

Fibromyalgia most commonly occurs in people who are otherwise perfectly healthy, with all organs, muscles, and joints in pristine condition. Fibromyalgia is not however exclusive to such healthy people. It can, and does occur, in many people who have a wide variety of other painful conditions alluded to earlier. It may occur in people who have any of the many forms of arthritis or spondylosis of the spine. It is also common in patients with well established Systemic Lupus. In such people it gives rise to the usual painful areas and fatigue. The development of fibromyalgia in such people can be easily missed. It may be regarded as a worsening of a pre existing disease and treated inappropriately. This is a common occurrence and it is a major reason why your doctor, rather than self-professed health gurus, should be consulted.

Less well recognised is the fact that the arrival of fibromyalgia has implications for pre-existing arthritis, for instance. Pain is the worst aspect of arthritis. With the onset of fibromyalgia the pain threshold is greatly lowered. This does not influence the activity of the arthritis itself.

However, because the sensitivity to pain is increased, the pain levels caused by the ongoing inflammation in the joints are also raised.

Many such people feel that the arthritis has got worse and increase their consumption of anti-inflammatory or pain-killing medications. This naturally proves to be of no help. All progress is stalled until the fibromyalgia component is recognised, dealt with appropriately and totally eradicated.

Exhaustion in FM

Exhaustion and fatigue are important and debilitating components of the fibromyalgia syndrome. They, like pain, must have a cause. It has already been suggested that exhaustion is present regardless of the time spent sleeping and that it is not abolished by sleep.

Therefore, if the *quantity* of sleep is in order there must be something the matter with the *quality* of the sleep itself. Sleep has a very important function in the maintenance of health and well being. Why else should nature dictate we spend one third of our lives in this state? Sleep replenishes body and soul. Sleep is not simply a 'lights out' situation. Neither is it a uniform state of the absence of consciousness, all through the night. It consists of various phases and stages, each with its own unique role in the restorative processes of the body and mind.

You are probably familiar with the term rapid eye movement (REM) sleep. There are many other stages of sleep in addition to this. These are collectively known as the non-REM stages. In many fibromyalgia sufferers an abnormal electrical activity of the brain occurs during one of these non-REM phases. This can be detected by electroencephalographic (EEG) tests. These tests are similar to electrical tests carried out on the heart by electrocardiographic (ECG) testing.

These electrical abnormalities disrupt the normal sleep pattern and while they may not interfere with the overall quantity of sleep, they do lessen the amount of time spent in the body-refreshing phase of sleep. The cause of exhaustion then is a sleep disorder that in simple terms damages sleep quality, rather than sleep quantity. This results in your waking up in the morning without your body being refreshed by the night's sleep.

This sleep can be described as being non-restorative in quality. It results in the question: *Do you wake up in the morning refreshed and restored by your sleep?* being one of the most important questions that must be put to the person who may have FM.

The exact abnormalities in sleep are poorly understood and current theories may have to be altered in time but the salient point is that poor sleep quality is an inherent part of fibromyalgia syndrome.

Again it can be appreciated that the complexity of the cause of the fatigue of fibromyalgia means that it is an entity that differs greatly from a tiredness one may have from the mere lack of sleep.

Pain-Fatigue link

It is not difficult to understand that poor sleep quality can give rise to chronic exhaustion. It can also be appreciated that a relative deficiency of pain suppressors can lessen the pain threshold to the extent that normal areas of the body register as being painful. It is a little more difficult to tie them together.

There are some chemicals in the brain that are thought to both modulate pain control, and exert a beneficial effect on the body-refreshing phase of sleep. It is thought that a deficiency of chemicals with these combined properties is the major biochemical cause of the pain and the fatigue. Different chemicals are being investigated and while some are showing promise, no particular one has been specifically identified though at any given time some chemicals are considered favourites for the role.

Currently the chemical serotonin is under a lot of investigation as it can influence both pain interpretation and sleep quality but many other chemicals, some as yet unidentified, most likely play major roles.

With regard to the pain-fatigue link of fibromyalgia, it is of great interest to note that in a research programme fibromyalgia syndrome was induced in healthy volunteers by subjecting them to selective sleep phase deprivation. Basically this involved buzzing them out of the body-refreshing phase of sleep, when this sleep phase became apparent on the EEG.

It resulted in many developing the symptoms of fibromyalgia. This indicates the critical role of sleep and also emphasises the relationship between fatigue and pain in fibromyalgia.

Current exciting developments in the field of chemical substances in the brain have not yet led to improved treatments but do give rise to cautious optimism. However, the understanding of the actions of the chemicals and of their exact role in FM is in its infancy. It should not result in anyone with fibromyalgia sitting back in the belief that a marvellous breakthrough has been made and that a cure is imminent. This cure, or external solution, is not at all imminent and if you want to get better you have much hard work to do. Success will ultimately depend on your ability to do this work.

Life with Fibromyalgia

Fibromyalgia is a most miserable condition to contend with. Each day has a dreary and debilitating sameness, though some may be that bit better or worse than average.

No day presents itself as a new day, with new opportunities. Each day starts with pain, stiffness, and fatigue. The stiffness and indeed the pain often ease after some hours. The resolution of the stiffness may be hastened by availing of a hot shower, a bath or a massage. Many have to use these methods to get started for the day.

The pain is, essentially, ever present. Many of the day's activities tend to aggravate the pain but generally not to the extent that any particular chores cannot be done.

Superimposed on the pain, stiffness, and physical discomfort, is the burden of exhaustion. Together these symptoms add considerably to the difficulties encountered in normal day-to-day living. This applies equally to occupations that involve physical work and those that involve mental work.

The majority of people feel exhausted on waking. Some are not too bad in the morning but tire early in the afternoon, regardless of activity. Even work that was greatly enjoyed, now becomes an onerous chore. Tasks that previously took very little out of you physically or mentally and which you would have no difficulty in dealing with, now are very draining. A day that would previously represent little of a challenge, now becomes a major obstacle course to the extent that you have to beat or fight your way through it.

Getting to the end of the day becomes an end in itself. It takes infinitely more out of you than it should to the extent that you are completely washed out and exhausted in the evening. The end of the day brings little reprieve. Because of the pain and exhaustion there is no enjoyment to be had from association with friends, family or children.

The irritability that often becomes a feature of fibromyalgia ensures that the feeling is mutual in many cases. You are not the person your family and friends once knew. What should be your happy relaxed period is simply not so, but is rather an extension of the day's difficulties.

Nothing is looked forward to. What was once joyful is now burdensome. Even children can be an effort to enjoy. Laughter seems beyond you: like your childhood, gone forever.

The difficulty in maintaining normal relationships with family and friends is a source of great tension for all people with fibromyalgia. A feeling of guilt often further compounds this. Leisure activities such as sports are generally abandoned. So also are normal social activities. This leads the person with fibromyalgia into a state of withdrawal and isolated misery. Hopelessness and misery are worsened by the knowledge that tomorrow, next week, and next month will bring nothing but more of the same.

What's so different?

It is true that many conditions give rise to pain and indeed a loss of general well-being. Again reference will be made to arthritis. However, people with arthritis have a tangible explanation for their symptoms. Even if the arthritis is severe and the associated disability is a great impingement to a normal life, there is an understanding as to why the situation is as it is.

The person with fibromyalgia will also feel afflicted physically. However, neither she nor indeed anyone she consults for help, can understand why, or give her a logical explanation for the state she is in. This makes the situation very difficult to cope with. The absence of abnormal results in blood tests and x-rays, can lead to doubt about the extent of her suffering in some doctors' minds. Patients with fibromyalgia detect these doubts. This leads to anger initially, but many subsequently doubt their own sanity and the validity of their symptoms.

Most people with fibromyalgia feel that doctors do not fully appreciate what they are saying. This serves to increases the sense of isolation. Therefore, the absence of an explanation for symptoms, the doubts as to whether anyone believes them, self doubt and sometimes guilt, all contrive to render fibromyalgia a more serious disorder, than many other diseases that the public view as being very serious.

Present-day medical knowledge is such that people with readily recognisable diseases are supported by the various medical systems that are in operation in all parts of the world, whether they be those in the western world, or in areas where technological advances are not so great. This supportive role applies not only to medical systems but also to people generally. Society still has a reservoir of sympathy for those it perceives to be physically ill. Concern and generally speaking a desire to help people who are ill remains a human characteristic. This may not appear to be much in its own right, but it does help to buttress the coping mechanisms of all people who have diseases that people generally understand.

As no one understands fibromyalgia, this sympathy, concern and empathy, sadly, is not available to its sufferers. Rather the attitude is that if there is something the matter then you should go to the system and get it fixed. Failure to go, take the treatment and declare yourself fit and act accordingly, indicates that the fault lies with you and that you are somehow a failure. In this respect you may well be your most ardent and severe critic.

Basically, if you have fibromyalgia, as opposed to any of the diseases that make the popularity ratings, you are on your own. It is a lonely place to be. Patients with a well-recognised and accepted disease visit a doctor and come away feeling much better if only for talking to him or her. This is a fact of life. They may have the added bonus of improved pain relief by virtue of a change of medication or more dramatically perhaps, by an injection into a painful joint.

People with fibromyalgia have none of this. Certainly they are not going to receive medication that makes any significant indentation in their symptoms or improves life quality in any way.

Neither indeed do they come away from meeting the doctor feeling better by virtue of the powers vested in all satisfactory consultations between patients and doctors. The bond or rapport between patient and physician is always good when both understand each other, and when the physician can at least recognise the disorder he or she is dealing with. This rapport is seldom soundly established in the case of fibromyalgia. Because the condition is poorly understood consultations are trying for both patient and physician and are often tense, uncomfortable affairs. You come away confused and sometimes hurt by the encounter.

Thus medical personnel, immediate friends, and society at large who are important allies of anyone with a recognised disease are not available to support you or to help you initially cope and later succeed in your efforts to get back to normal health.

A distinction is being made here between your trusted family doctor, who wants you to become well, and a great variety of others in whose best interest it lies that you remain ill. There are many therapists of various descriptions that give ridiculous diagnoses to people with fibromyalgia. All of these diagnoses seem to make sense and all the treatments cost money. Such treatments also seem to be never ending. Even the most intelligent of people go for these false treatments. The usual reason given by people with fibromyalgia for availing of what are patently illogical treatments is that 'you will do anything when you are in pain'.

Another reason is that spurious alternative practitioners will always give you a clear-cut black and white diagnosis. Their certainty, while utterly false, gives the forlorn person with FM something to cling to. Here you will receive culturally acceptable diagnoses such as having bones or discs out or a strain of the sacro-iliac joint. Other nonsense that is advocated is that you may be suffering from fungal infections, too much acid in the blood or allergies to various substances. These false diagnoses are often backed up by fraudulent tests.

One way or the other you continue to avail of their spurious treatments until such time as you can afford them no longer, or else realise that they are good for nothing. It is easy for orthodox medicine to take the high moral ground but if its efforts were more successful or even if it was capable of establishing a proper relationship with the fibromyalgia sufferer, then the need for sham treatments would decline rapidly.

In Canada and the USA where fibromyalgia is common and in Britain where CFS is very frequently diagnosed there are now added problems. It seems that FM was being tolerated as a real problem and a real source of disability until such time as it became greatly damaging to the profits of some interests. Efforts are now underway to discredit FM and to portray such people as malingerers or psychological mis-fits. This is bound to have a further demoralising effect on a down-trodden group of suffering people. As stated earlier, there are some people in Canada and the United States who do seek financial and other gains, by feigning symptoms of FM. These people are doing untold damage to genuine sufferers.

At the end of the day it is possible that big money will win out and that FM will again by neglected, but by then you will be better!

However, the question of disability and the socio-economic consequences of FM are not an issue here. This book is about getting better, so if it is successful, then long-term disability should not be an issue.

This is written for genuine sufferers and if you are still with me, it is reasonable to assume you are in this category.

Many factors conspire to make fibromyalgia a most miserable condition to have. Indeed any experienced doctor can view people in the waiting room of a rheumatology clinic and pick out those who have fibromyalgia. Most of the arthritis patients will have hope in their faces. The person with fibromyalgia emanates a palpable tension, born of the fact that she knows the doctor will not fully understand what she is talking about, that her tablets will be changed from one colour to another without any benefit and that the whole process will be repeated next visit.

In the period of confusion that prevails before the diagnosis is made and properly understood, some people with fibromyalgia will relate to medical personnel that they want a specific diagnosis: 'Tell me I have arthritis, cancer, or even multiple sclerosis'. What they are really saying is that they want a diagnosis, no matter how serious, that is understood by the public at large and more especially by friends. They feel it will somehow lessen their isolation and liberate them from their prison where they are not accepted as sick, and yet are very unwell.

The response to treatment is another factor that is different for the person with fibromyalgia. Arthritis victims get some reprieve from treatment. If they are having a bad spell they may get temporary ease from increasing their painkillers.

If they wish to go out for a night's entertainment then a few steroid tablets may allow them to do so, within reason.

Such a temporary reprieve is not available for fibromyalgia sufferers. Tablets make no difference. On the contrary fibromyalgia has the capacity to keep you totally in its control regardless of what efforts you make. Fibromyalgia dominates your life in a manner in which no other condition can. All tasks, chores, sporting and social activities are undertaken in reference to your ability to cope with them and in deference to their ability at times to completely debilitate you. If you wish to go out for the evening your ability to do so will be determined by fibromyalgia and not by you, or by others.

You are the prisoner. Fibromyalgia is your warden. You have no rights, only occasional privileges at the utter discretion of fibromyalgia.

Other factors

Psychological distress is very common in fibromyalgia. The most common manifestation of this is irritability and mood swings. The sufferer experiences constant fatigue, an inability to enjoy life, and of course the feeling of isolation. There is also a sense of injustice in that you can get no reprieve from symptoms no matter what steps you take and no matter to whom you reach for help.

There is the sense of not being believed in your suffering. You certainly do not want sympathy but you would appreciate some empathy from those most close to you and something more from professional helpers.

The more tablets, more medical investigations, more physical therapies, more senseless physical manipulations or placebo or sham treatments that are given, the more intense your awareness that you are no longer the person you once were. You have the feeling that your whole world is spiralling out of your control. Frustration and inappropriate guilt are felt in various mixes.

The end result is irritability, anxiety, anger, or a feeling of depression. This often manifests itself in hostility to friends and loved ones, the very people who should be your best allies and indeed would be in the event of your suffering a more recognised and more understandable disease. Friends do not call around so much. Loved ones are hurt, alienated or feel useless and frustrated.

In essence fibromyalgia affects not just the immediate victim but also those most close to them. Social life is often avoided: home life can become fraught with tension. Emotional upset becomes a feature of your fibromyalgia syndrome.

Irritable bowel symptoms, discomfort passing urine, and areas of tingling or numbness are features already mentioned as occurring in some people. These too must have an explanation.

Such features most likely have the same basis as does the symptom of pain. Just as the pain threshold is reduced so also is the threshold for awareness of symptoms other than pain. With regard to bowel symptoms the level of awareness of normal intestinal functional activity is raised. Normally such sensations do not register in the consciousness. However, they do in people with FM.

The point here again is that sensations you interpret as unpleasant are not indicative of a disease process but are indicative of a disorder of pain and other sensory processing due to the various chemical imbalances in brain tissue or fluids.

The same applies to the pins and needles and feeling of swelling in and about the joints. Some people with fibromyalgia do tend to have actual swelling of the fingers to the extent that rings may be tight and may have to be removed. This is detectable on examination and is an objective finding rather than a subjective complaint.

It is known as idiopathic edema. In simple language this is fluid retention in the absence of heart disease or kidney disease. It has a different origin than does the pain, but it relates to increased sensitivity to the normal hormones that in this case regulate fluid balance.

Cognitive dysfunction consisting of impaired memory, difficulties in concentration and with mental arithmetic, is complained of by many with fibromyalgia.

However, in some surveys when subject to direct testing, people with fibromyalgia were not nearly so bad as they thought they were. It can be suggested that you have so much on your mind and are in such a state of perpetual turmoil, that in day-to-day living ordinary events do not register as comprehensively as they should, while in the more relaxed setting of a test environment, people perform better. All people, in practical terms, know that it is difficult to concentrate or remember small things when they are 'bothered' by other matters and no doubt the presence of constant pain also does not help. This is but another manifestation of the all-pervasiveness of FM in your life.

Standard Investigations and Treatment

Fibromyalgia is readily diagnosed on the basis of the typical symptom profile and the physical findings. The symptoms are very distinctive ones. The absence of a response to treatment is not mentioned as being very important in any of the publications on fibromyalgia. In spite of this, it is one of the most critically important of all features. Basically if people can say that they get good relief from standard painkillers it is almost certain that they don't have fibromyalgia. Therefore the symptoms are the most important factors in arriving at a diagnosis.

Much is made of the physical findings. The only physical finding is tenderness to touch. This, however, is not a clear-cut black and white objective finding in the way swelling or reduced mobility of a joint in arthritis would be. Far too much is made of the number and location of tender points, especially in countries where disability payments are made for FM. The inadequacies of the ACR criteria are also partly responsible for this.

The general inadequacies of blood tests and other investigations have already been established. Undue emphasis on 'tests' is encountered in hi-tech clinics and this is to the detriment of the time-honoured art of being able to talk to the patient.

Far too often when the patient refuses to get better, it is directly or indirectly implied that it's all in her head. This really is the fault of doctors who cannot cope with people not responding to their treatments as well as they think they should.

However, with increasing medical sophistication many of the wiser doctors are paradoxically becoming more aware of their limitations and are better able to cope with apparent failure than they might have been years ago.

Current treatments

Medical treatments for fibromyalgia are ineffective. If they were satisfactory then there would be no need to read a book such as this. They are all of little or no benefit and the fact that they are still used widely is a reflection of the poor general understanding of fibromyalgia.

Persistence with treatments, in spite of the fact that it is obvious that they are useless, shows how medical personnel (whether orthodox or alternative), need to keep treating even when the treatment is serving no purpose. It also shows how all people who believe themselves to be diseased need to consume medical products of some sort or another.

The usual story is that the patient attends orthodox medicine, though in recent years there is a greater tendency to go to various alternative practitioners, much vaunted in media productions, mainly directed at women.

Various painkillers or anti-inflammatory medications are given for the pain. When these make no difference, physical therapy is often employed. Some aspects of this can be temporarily soothing, such as the application of heat or gentle massage.

Many of the treatments used in physical therapy clinics have no more than a placebo effect. By placebo effect is meant that any treatment will have some beneficial effect if a patient believes in it.

Worse still many people with fibromyalgia are told that the tender areas represent muscle spasm. They do nothing of the sort. In fact, spasm is not a cause of pain in any medical condition outside of tetanus. This mis-diagnosis would not matter except for the fact that it often leads to the use of muscle relaxants or worse still, tranquillisers.

Again, because it is believed by some that there is disease or micro-spasm in the painful areas, these regions are often injected with local anaesthetic with or without added steroid in the hope of alleviating symptoms. These sometimes prove to be of very transient benefit but make no difference overall. This particular line of treatment was availed of by this author many years ago but it has now been all but fully abandoned as it has proved to be of no significant benefit.

That medical intervention is ineffective is not just an assertion of this booklet, but is recognised as such in the publications of all the leading clinical researchers in the field of fibromyalgia and of course by the FM population itself.

The failure of treatments is frequently blamed on some psychological aberration on the part of the patient. This occasionally leads to the administration of tranquillisers or anti-depressants.

Some patients go so far as to attend specialist pain clinics. This involves encounters with physical therapists, psychologists, psychiatrists, occupational therapists, behavioural therapists and medical practitioners in various other fields.

Fibromyalgia people in such circumstances feel as though they are being taken over and many quickly recoil from such institutions. Some pain clinics genuinely try to help but some others are of a very poor standard.

At this stage rock bottom has been reached, and social and family life is often in tatters. The alternative trail is then embarked on. There is no question here of a practitioner saying, 'I don't know!' A diagnosis is always made and presented with utmost conviction. Such certainty is most reassuring for the patient and hope rises.

However, it perishes on the rocks of such groundless diagnoses as bones or discs being out, one leg being longer than the other, sacro-iliac strain, or mal-alignment of the jaw or some segments of the spine.

Patients will be assured by the enthusiastic and plausible practitioner who will then proceed to make your back or neck click. Of course you want to believe that something has been put back, and of course you will be assured that it is.

Nothing of the sort has happened. These treatments, if you can tolerate them, do seem to help temporarily. The help is not due to any beneficial alteration in your spine, but to the already mentioned placebo effect. These treatments also can be dangerous and there have been reports of strokes and deaths after neck manipulations. At any rate, they have no long-term benefit and are fortunately eventually abandoned by the person with FM.

These nonsensical treatments are bad enough but worse still, many people with fibromyalgia are told that their problems relate to an ongoing viral infection or the after-effects of such an infection. This ongoing viral theory is indeed bad news. If it was just another piece of misguided speculation it would be no worse than any other. If a person believes she has a continuing viral problem she believes that she has an actual disease. She also believes that it is then the responsibility of a doctor to make her better.

Medicine cannot cure fibromyalgia and it is not the responsibility of any doctor to treat a person with fibromyalgia as though it were a standard disease model or to give her any hope that therapies will make a significant difference. In fact, it is the treatment of FM as a standard disease that has led in the past to the abysmal failure of all therapies.

The person who believes she has a virus or the after-effects of a virus, believes that she has no responsibility for her own well-being; this, as will be explained, is a serious error. Studies have shown that people who believe that a virus has caused their problem and who feel a cure should be provided for them, do badly overall.

The quest for a cure becomes a preoccupation. It becomes an end in itself and the patient single-mindedly keeps ploughing on, while all around, her world is falling apart. It does eventually dawn on her that she is getting nowhere.

Modern medicine has its good and bad points. It has achieved many good things. People today rarely die of appendicitis or meningitis, if treated in time. Neither do women die in child birth. The down side of modern medicine is that all people are conditioned to believe that medicine has the answer to everything. Thus the patient with fibromyalgia embarks on her affair with medicine with a high level of expectation and seeks a total cure. The level of expectation, often fuelled by the medical profession itself, is outrageously high. When medicine fails the fibromyalgia patient, as it inevitably does, the person blames herself. This newly-acquired guilt adds only further to the burden. Hopelessness now prevails even more.

Medicine, whether orthodox or alternative, is of no help to the person with fibromyalgia. On the contrary the sufferer benefits the various practitioners, in that she is a consummate consumer of medical products. In effect, many afflicted with fibromyalgia become converted into long-term patients, addicted to the various treatments on offer from countless sources.

Orthodox and alternative medicine are equally detrimental to the person with fibromyalgia. They both tell you that you are diseased. They both tell you that you can do little for yourself.

They both wrongly tell you that you are a patient and that your only hope of salvation is to purchase their products for a price. They both undermine your inherent ability to overcome the disorder. They are both equally patronising and when you acquire a full understanding of what it is that ails you, you will clearly see this assertion to be a fact.

Treatment failures

Any person with fibromyalgia will derive very little benefit from the currently available treatments. Why do they not work? Why does an anti-inflammatory drug, whether of the steroidal or non-steriodal variety, make no difference? What is it about the pain of fibromyalgia that makes it so different? An anti-inflammatory can work only when there is a painful inflammatory disease. Fibromyalgia as explained is not in this category. In essence, there is nothing for anti-inflammatories to do, and nothing they can do except perhaps upset your stomach.

The pain and tenderness does not indicate that there is a disease process in the painful area but, rather, that the pain threshold is reduced to the extent that a totally normal area of the body registers as being painful and often exquisitely painful. This can be quite difficult to fully comprehend. Some people cannot understand how a very painful area is not a site of diseased or inflamed tissue. This misconception is easy to empathise with but even so it is one you will have to come to terms with.

The cause of the pain in fibromyalgia is a relative deficiency of the body's own pain modifiers. These are not anti-inflammatories or analgesics (painkillers). In fact the chemicals that control pain threshold in no way relate to anti-inflammatories. Therefore consuming anti-inflammatories serves no significant practical purpose. If you do not understand this now, you are at a very serious disadvantage.

People with FM, by and large, are very intolerant of medications and frequently report that even low doses of commonly used over-the-counter (OTC) preparations cause side effects. This is actually to their advantage as it renders their minds more open to a non-medicinal road to recovery. Furthermore FM sufferers are by and large reluctant tablet takers and sick patient status does not rest easily with them.

Steroid tablets are basically very strong anti-inflammatories but, for all their potency in many diseases, they are not effective, at all treatment in FM. Ordinary painkillers also have very little effect generally, though some people find they provide a little transient benefit.

Surprisingly, heat, such as may be procured by lying in hot water or by applying more direct heat, can be very soothing, if only for a while. Theories abound as to why this should be so, but if it helps it should be availed of as it certainly is not going to do any harm.

Massage is soothing but then again massage is only the application of heat, though this simple fact is shrouded in mystery in various physical therapy clinics. Massage is often given on the mistaken premise that it is breaking down taut bands of tissue. This is but more of the nonsense that people with FM have to contend with.

Massage does not break down adhesions, or loosen out or soothe taut fibrositic nodules, or break up the sweet-sounding pain-spasm-pain cycle (an irrational and senseless term that does not stands up to scrutiny but continues to be widely used).

Various creams and rubs are widely availed of. These make little or no difference at all, but by and large are harmless. Other medications and treatment strategies are widely availed of but are not of much value and will be discussed later.

At any rate, if you have got this far it is to be hoped that you will persist with the more self-reliant route that will be advocated.

Fatigue treatment

Fatigue is a major feature of fibromyalgia. Efforts at its eradication are indeed justified. However, to date, an effective fatigue treatment has eluded researchers and practitioners.

Many FM sufferers believe that their fatigue is due to the fact that their sleep is disturbed by periods of wakefulness brought about by pain. This is not so. All people wake from their sleep many times during the night and quickly return to sleep. The fact that they actually wake up does not register with the vast majority of people.

This is not the case for anyone who has pain. Each moment of being awake registers clearly in the consciousness. It is for this reason that many people with FM insist that their fatigue is caused by broken sleep that in turn is due to pain.

Research has shown that people with FM do wake up a little more often at night than other people, but the difference is very little.

This slight increase in night-time wakefulness cannot account for your fatigue. People with medical problems try to rationalise everything and it is often very hard to convince FM sufferers that their fatigue is not due to broken sleep. It is sometimes equally difficult to convince people with a disc protrusion in their necks that it was not caused by a draught from an open door or car window.

The problem with sleep relates not to its quantity, nor to its being broken, but rather to its quality. In fibromyalgia people do not get proper undisturbed non-REM sleep. This is the body-refreshing phase of sleep. Therefore they wake up not refreshed or restored by sleep. As the disorder is one of quality, not quantity, it therefore makes no difference how long a time you spend sleeping. Evidence that this is the case is provided by accounts given by true insomniacs. There are people who have been observed to truly spend very little time in sleep. They do not have any symptoms that even remotely resemble the fatigue or the pain of FM.

From this it can be deduced also that there is nothing to be gained at all from spending extra time in bed especially during the day; this is a mistake many people with fibromyalgia used to make in the past. This applied even more so to those labelled CFS.

Likewise, sedatives, otherwise known as sleeping tablets, offer little benefit. These help you stay asleep for a longer period than you might without them. They do not address the fundamental problem of sleep quality and really have no useful role to play in overcoming the real causes of the condition.

Spurious Treatments

Fibromyalgia is not a serious disease insofar as it does not shorten life. As treatments are so ineffective and as sufferers of FM are so desperate to get something to alleviate their abject misery, there is no shortage of people providing products that they claim will alleviate symptoms and cure fibromyalgia. Unfortunately, while these treatments are utterly irrational, people frequently avail of them. People with fibromyalgia are not unique in this respect. Arthritis and cancer patients will go from one end of the world to the other, in order to avail of treatments that are expensive, false, useless, and often deliberately misleading.

With regard to FM there are a host of treatments promoted on the open market. Sometimes these are promoted as natural health products and false pseudo-scientific evidence is provided for their usefulness. Often these claims are backed up by people who allegedly had FM saying they were cured. Other sufferers are told they have fungal infections and are given anti-fungal drugs or ridiculous diets.

Others are subject to unscientific testing and sometimes are advised to go on exclusion diets. Various spinal and sacro-iliac manipulations are in the same category insofar as being useful is concerned. Many of these spurious tests and treatments cost alot in time wasted, and in actual money spent. Their main disadvantage lies in the fact that they convince you that you are diseased and in need of treatment for that disease. They lead to a further delay in accepting the true nature of your disorder and they weaken your resolve to get better by your own efforts. Indeed they specifically imply that it is not within your power to beat FM without purchasing these products.

Such products will be ever increasing in number and there are already too many of them to list in this book. In addition to this you will frequently come under pressure from friends to avail of them even while you may be going along with the management plan outlined here. Rest assured that if there was a useful treatment for FM it would be a very major breakthrough and would be widely covered in all rheumatology textbooks and periodicals, and your doctor would only be too glad to provide you with it.

If you are a victim of FM the situation is bad enough without your being subject to ridiculously expensive and sometimes physically dangerous treatments.

What Causes Fibromyalgia?

Fibromyalgia represents a breakdown in the normal pain and sleep control mechanisms, resulting in pain, fatigue, and all the other associated symptoms. Something in turn must give rise to these breakdowns.

No-one knows what this is and there-in lies the major mystery of fibromyalgia. Scientists are attempting to find out what biochemical abnormalities may be causing the poor sleep and poor pain tolerance but no one is asking why these biochemical abnormalities are occurring in the first place.

So what, if substance P may be present in excessive amounts in the brain fluid, or serotonin levels may be a bit low in the brain tissue. So what, if the production of hormones by the pituitary gland (part of the brain) may be somewhat abnormal in response to various stimulation tests. The real question that needs to be addressed and answered is, Why?

No one, it appears, knows the answer and it is not clear if the question has ever been addressed properly.

The author has his own views as to the cause of FM, views with which other people may or may not agree. People with fibromyalgia have certain characteristics and personality traits that may provide very important clues as to the true solution to this fundamental problem.

The most striking feature is that most people with FM are intense, meticulous, perfectionist type personalities (IMPs). Others could be described as worriers. Everything they do must be perfect. All must be done by themselves. If not, then nothing is done to their own exacting standards. It irks them to see others do what they know they can do so much better themselves. They cannot delegate. They set their own standards and they are their own harshest critics. By and large they are infinitely more intolerant of their own shortcomings than they are of similar failings in others.

They are more than willing workers. As such, they take on more than their share of responsibility at work. They are prized workers. Others, not of a similar nature, let them go ahead. In most cases potential sufferers take the extra burdens on themselves. In some instances, it is dumped on them.

Those who might be described as easy-going, laid-back people do not get fibromyalgia. In my experience this statement is sacrosanct.

It is the contention of this book that people with fibromyalgia take too much on themselves and that the excess burden eventually leads to the breakdown in pain and sleep control systems.

It is too convenient to suggest this is a stress-related disorder. To suggest this is to wrongly apply a debased and overused cliché to something of a far different origin.

It also implies some type of psychological failure to cope with the stresses and strains of life which in my view are not at all pertinent to fibromyalgia.

In this book it is strongly advocated that people of a particular personality prototype take too much on, for far too long a period of time and that this in turn leads directly or indirectly to the breakdown in the normal sleep and pain control mechanisms of the body. Only people of a certain personality type are thus susceptible to the development of the disorder and there is a tendency for it to run in families.

Whatever about this being broadly accepted it is suggested that you as an individual will make no progress in your conflict unless you not only accept what is written here, but also endorse it fully.

In order to make progress you will also have to accept that what you have is in fact fibromyalgia. It is no good accepting the diagnosis just because some doctor believes you have it.

It is the experience of this author that fibromyalgia virtually never occurs after a single specific physical or psychologically traumatic event, or that the syndrome might be so induced in an already susceptible individual. In the United States, in particular, the experience of many genuine workers in the area of fibromyalgia is at variance with this. This author recognises and respects their views.

This book is based on the author's personal experience and its aim is to help you recover normal health and vitality. A singular effort is made throughout to avoid side issues as the road to recovery is the same regardless of whether or not a single event may have precipitated the onset or worsened an already pre-existing degree of fibromyalgia.

You will know from what you have just read if you have fibromyalgia or not. You have to see for yourself that you suffer the effects of FM. The most important first stage on the road to recovery is accepting that your problem is truly FM, based on the account of the symptom profile that has been presented here. From the doctor's perspective one of the most hopeful indicators of a satisfactory outcome is that people with FM will report that they feel that what is written here could have been written about them personally.

Psychological factors

There have been many studies of a psychological nature carried out on people with fibromyalgia, and none have indicated any psychological abnormality as being relative to its cause. Of course, if one wishes to consider the personality prototype that I regard as being uniquely susceptible to fibromyalgia as being a disease state, then that is their right. Humans are not personality clones. There are many different personality types as any school teacher, for instance, can readily identify in the classroom. There is no ideal and the individual variations are but expressions of the heterogeneity of the human condition.

Fibromyalgia people resent any suggestions of psychological factors playing a role in their condition and it is easy to understand why. This however, can be overdone.

Far too much energy is devoted towards eradicating any such suggestions by people with fibromyalgia and by spokespersons for organisations that represent them. This amounts to nothing more than the expenditure of energy that would be better channelled in other directions.

Paranoia about the suggestion that psychological factors are important is a silly and self-defeating position to assume. In the first instance it betrays an ignorance of the fact that there is virtually no disease state in which psychological factors do not play a role, either in the manifestation of the disease itself, or in one's ability to cope with it. People with psoriasis or colitis do not seem to have any problem accepting that psychological factors play a role in their disease expression. They know that if they are in good form and at peace with themselves and their environment, their disease is less likely to be active than when they are under a lot of pressure.

What of people with acute heart failure whose lungs are flooded with water and who are in fact drowning? The terrible distress of these people is immediately relieved by morphine. Their breathing eases and they can actually speak, which many in the acute phase are too breathless or exhausted to do.

This improvement occurs in spite of the fact that x-rays reveal that their lungs are still full of water. While morphine plays a number of roles in such a situation, its most immediate benefit is that it lessens anxiety and stress.

These points are mentioned in the hope that spokespersons for those with fibromyalgia and indeed the victims themselves will avoid misdirecting energy in deriding the efforts of excellent psychologists who have made significant contributions to the understanding of fibromyalgia.

All contributions should be graciously accepted. The real sadness, however, lies in the fact that people with fibromyalgia seem to be on the defensive and tend to believe that the physical validity of their suffering is lessened by any such suggestions. Education and knowledge are most important aids on your journey to normal health. Closing your mind to what you may not wish to hear is counter-productive.

While accepting that psychological weakness does not play a role in the genesis of fibromyalgia, it is true that tenseness, irritability, and mood changes do eventually become a major part of the syndrome. Any person who is in chronic pain, who is chronically exhausted, experiencing no respite from treatment, who has received no tangible explanation for the condition, who feels that others doubt her credibility, and who sees no light at the end of the tunnel, will be very tense and uptight.

It is not surprising that many are regarded as being depressed. People with fibromyalgia, especially those who have suffered for a long time, can look haggard, miserable, and older than their years.

Some, however, remain looking perfectly healthy. They will relate that they are fed up with being told by others, how well they look, as though such statements were casting doubts on their illness or their degree of suffering. It is disappointing that they should feel this way. To be told 'You look well' (whether true or not) gives most people a boost. Not so for those with fibromyalgia who read something else into it, often very wrongly. What people with FM read into this compliment is that the person making the statement is really saying that, because she is the picture of health, nothing could possibly be wrong with her.

Unlike most other medical conditions the person with fibromyalgia rarely reaches a state of equilibrium with her illness. The arthritic copes with his pain and disability. The amputee gets on without his missing limb and often resents being regarded as handicapped. The person with fibromyalgia by contrast never comes to terms with her disorder and because of this suffers all the more. It should be clear at this stage that there are complexities to FM that do not apply to common disease states. It can also be seen that the efforts of anyone to equate FM with other common disease states are misdirected and while they persist they are not helping anyone with FM.

Other Suggested Causes of FM

There are many who will not accept what is written here and who put forward quite a numbers of theories on what they believe to be the cause of fibromyalgia. Some of these theories are compatible with those espoused here, while some of them are not at all.

Psychological theories

There are many practitioners who cannot appreciate that a person can have a physical illness, if a physical examination and the appropriate laboratory and radiological tests are normal. This is an understandable fact in newly-qualified interns. However, such an attitude is not acceptable from more experienced practitioners. Anyone can appreciate the frustration doctors will feel when they are doing their best, and yet cannot come up with what they consider a tangible and real diagnosis. This frustration is added to when the patient's symptoms do not respond to the treatments administered. Such doctors may fall prey to suggestions that fibromyalgia is not a real physical entity at all.

However, they fail to appreciate the subtle difference between a disorder and a disease and they fail to appreciate that the former often presents much more formidable problems both for themselves and their patient. They believe, or are led to believe, that their patient must have some psychological disorder that renders the stresses of their lives too much for them to bear. They believe that their patient wishes to assume what is referred to as the sick-patient role.

People who assume the sick-patient role consciously or sub-consciously develop symptoms that suggest to themselves and to others that they are ill. Such people expect others to give unto them the role granted to the sick person in society. They demand the concern of others and relief from their normal social responsibilities. It is further suggested that it suits these people better to have a physical rather than a psychological or psychiatric illness. In simple language, it is suggested that the assumption of the sick-role is a suitable cop-out for some people under pressure. By the same token people with genuine FM could suggest that such a belief represents a simple cop-out for a doctor who is unable to cope with a patient's condition.

There is no doubt that people who adopt the sick role exist, and have assumed the symptoms of many well-defined illnesses. The sick role allows them to cop out or to abdicate their working and social responsibilities. In a way, it becomes a solution to life's problems, although not a satisfactory one.

Could fibromyalgia be a manifestation of this psychological disorder? I suggest that it could not, and I present a few reasons for this opinion.

If a person wants to be regarded as sick it would be very difficult to conceive a more tactless choice than fibromyalgia.

People with fibromyalgia may initially receive some sympathy but this frequently turns to annoyance and rejection. People with other illnesses have bonds with loved ones strengthened, whereas the fibromyalgia person becomes very isolated.

The person with a feigned illness always chooses well recognised clear-cut symptoms, easily described; symptoms that closely resemble those complained of by patients with back problems, heart or lung disease, abdominal pain or headaches.

People with fibromyalgia cannot even begin to explain how they feel.

Psychological-problem-people feel believed or else they cut out of the game. The fibromyalgia sufferer is genuinely trapped and has nowhere to go. Society does not empathise with her or support her. Neither does the sufferer find support from the medical world. None of this applies to the person who successfully achieves the sick-role by assuming symptoms of other disorders.

Overall people with a psychological disorder will have what appears to be real and understandable symptoms compatible with their social background, education, and intelligence. They are very much at ease with their new role and benefit greatly from it. The fibromyalgia person presents a profile of symptoms devoid of logic to herself and others. If fibromyalgia is a falsehood, it is a real dumb choice. The victim never gets anymore than the briefest moment of sympathy.

This author practises in a society where fibromyalgia is not widely appreciated, is not recognised as an illness that is associated with disability and is not financially gainful in any way.

There is no conceivable secondary gain and yet it is a most common disorder. In some disorders such as "whiplash" where there can be secondary gain it is suggested that learned behaviour gives rise to the symptoms.

That cannot apply to FM in countries where people by and large have no knowledge of the symptom profile of FM and where the vast majority of sufferers never heard of it before it was diagnosed in their own case. In all such countries people with FM have exactly the same symptoms in spite of having no contact with other sufferers of FM.

Authors in the United States are mindful of the fact that some people claim to have symptoms that would be compatible with fibromyalgia for secondary financial gain. It has to be accepted that there is a logical basis for some to feign the symptoms of fibromyalgia, where there is the potential for such gain.

This book, however, is for you and not for them. It is this author's experience that FM uncommonly leads to very lengthy periods off work and that the person's sole interest always lies in getting better.

If fibromyalgia is a modern day cop-out, why was it described back in 1904 in the *British Medical Journal*? How do children with fibromyalgia fit in with this convenient theory? If fibromyalgia had a basis in hysteria, then why are there no cultural differences in its expression throughout the world? People of all different cultural, educational, religious and ethnic backgrounds complain of exactly the same symptoms. In fact, far and away the best description I have ever encountered of the symptoms of fibromyalgia has been in Arabic. In a busy rheumatology clinic in a very rural area in a Middle Eastern Country, fibromyalgia was astonishingly common.

The presenting symptoms were virtually always *Coo Lou Alam, Cool Ohmree Thaban*; the most direct English translation of which is *All is pain, all my essence is tired*. These people did not speak English and they had no access to western world culture or media. They had no concept of FM nor, indeed, did they have a specific name for it in their own language. Social contact among women in that culture was minimal. Secondary gain was out of the question and their suffering was palpable. Needless to say, they also did not respond to treatments.

At the end of the last century hysteria was a very common condition though no doubt many with genuine diseases were wrongly labelled as such by doctors whose stupidity would shock even the most fatuous of today's exponents of medical arrogance.

Most of you will at one time or another have seen the dramatic fainting scenes of many of the old black and white films. All the drama was conjured up for secondary gain. There are now assertions from some quarters that the history of hysteria has gone from paralysis in the last century, to fatigue today.

This is a simple cop-out for those doctors who have never encountered or appreciated the real suffering of people with FM. The practising hysterics of the last century delightfully accommodated themselves to their devastating paralysis and seemingly, if the films are to be believed, looked even more angelic than ever. Again, if the films are to be taken at a reasonable amount of face value, it would appear that the infinite majority of hysterics were female.

This is so much in contrast to today's fibromyalgia sufferers who so clearly are at their wits end, so distraught and sometimes so bedraggled and so different to what they were before they became afflicted. In the last century people found hysterics endearing and charming. Today people with FM are often regarded as a pain in the neck by many people providing health care.

If hysteria is the basis of the pain and the fatigue then women certainly have changed over the years. While one might accept this, surely one cannot suggest that they have become so stupid as to assume the trappings of a disorder that will gain for them only contempt.

Stress aspects

Stress is part of life. It is perhaps a greater factor in life today than in former times. The world has changed more in the last 40 years than maybe it did in the previous two thousand. Many of the certainties of the past such as job security, and more significantly the guarantee of financial sufficiency if one was prepared to work hard, have now gone. Today there is an increasing emphasis on self sufficiency and personal development. Assertiveness has become a euphemism for one's ability to use others for one's own immediate benefit. We live in an adversarial system, a system that might have a well documented and honourable place in a court of law, but whose benefits have yet to be confirmed in day-to-day human life.

Nothing is certain; security is a thing of the past. Individuals now have to fend for themselves in isolation as opposed to participating in a community. This has all come about rather quickly and no one knows whether it is for the better or not.

Could FM possibly be the body's way of rejecting the mental anguish most people (apart from the privileged few) must be going through at least occasionally? Again, the answer is not known. However, stress alone cannot account for the development of FM. If stress alone could account for the development of, and continuing manifestations of FM, then why is it so commonly confined to the personality type already described as being so predisposed?

People predisposed to the ill effects of stress develop many disorders such as alcoholism, but certainly most doctors' experience with people with FM is that the incidence of substance abuse is very much lower than average. Likewise people with FM are very rare doctors-attendees until FM arrives on the scene.

People of the FM personality do tend to take too much on and as such they shoulder more than their fair share of the stresses in their environment. For that reason it can appear at first sight that stress may be the cause of their disorder. It is not as simple as this even though many would conveniently like to regard it as such.

In this book it is postulated that people with FM are, by nature, people who take too much on and the disturbance of the sleep pattern and pain control mechanisms with the subsequent development of the symptoms of FM is the price they pay for this.

People of a different nature will not generally endeavour to take too much on, and if stress interferes with their physical well-being it will do so in many different ways, clearly distinguishable from, and in no way related to, the symptoms of FM.

If stress is the major factor then psychologists, stress management courses and of course the various gurus idolised by middle-class columnists in the media, would have some element of success in dealing with it. They have none.

FM is very different to a mere physical response to stress as will be clear from the recommended lines of overcoming it. The end result of this book will be determined by your success in achieving normal health and perhaps when you are fully recovered, you can have your own say and put forward your own views. Indeed you may become a person who will in time be able to help other people, help them not to live with FM but rather live without it which is your present goal and which distinguishes this book from virtually all others that are produced to help you live well in spite of the symptoms of FM.

Hormonal changes

There are changes in the levels of some hormones in people who have fibromyalgia. The glands that are involved in the production of these hormones are primarily the hypothalamus, pituitary and adrenal.

While these changes have been documented, it is not suggested that they cause any of the symptoms of FM.

All of these glands are sensitive to stress, pain and fatigue. In this case, the term stress refers to that which an animal might be under when experiencing threat or danger. The hormones of these glands are linked up with the fear, flight and fight reactions that we attribute to animals under threat. These hormonal changes in humans with fibromyalgia are more likely secondary to the fatigue and chronic pain of fibromyalgia rather than primary factors in the cause of the disorder.

Which ever way you look at it, the various hormonal changes that have been detected in some people with FM are not in conflict with what is written here, but any suggestions that they are major factors in its development or expression, certainly are.

Likewise, there are no significant changes in female hormone levels that might go anyway towards explaining why women are so susceptible to the development of FM.

Changes in brain blood flow

Modern x-rays have detected some changes in blood flow to some parts of the brains of people with fibromyalgia. However, these changes are not unique to fibromyalgia and what their significance is, if any, remains to be determined. Many with FM who do not, and who will not understand their disorder want to believe that these findings are a major breakthrough. While of interest they are nothing of the sort and if undue reliance is placed upon them by you, then you are missing out on this opportunity to get well. Messing about while waiting for medicine to cure you is futile.

Depression

It would be very convenient if it could be shown that depression was the root cause of the symptoms of the fibromyalgia syndrome. Virtually all studies, no matter how great the intent to ensure the highest standards of protocol and avoid bias, are to some extent flawed.

However, what studies are available indicate that depression is not a cause of fibromyalgia and that it does not become a significant component of the syndrome later. People with FM can have serious depression as can people without the syndrome.

It is true that many people with fibromyalgia are utterly miserable. It is also true that many standard questionnaires that are used to diagnose depression may indicate that some people with fibromyalgia are depressed. However, these questionnaires are entirely unsuitable for people who are in chronic pain. It is no wonder that people with fibromyalgia will answer many depression questionnaires in the affirmative as they are in pain, misery, and in a state of constant exhaustion. It is for this reason that many are wrongly labelled depressed.

If depression was a causative factor or indeed a significant part of the syndrome in the majority of cases then there would be a substantial improvement after an appropriate treatment period with anti-depressant drugs or perhaps psychotherapy. There is no such response.

In fact it is quite amazing that people with fibromyalgia do not develop a considerable degree of reactive depression in response to the way they are regarded and in response to so much of the negative publicity people with the condition receive in some parts of the world.

People writing about fibromyalgia, with or without the backing of self-help groups, are often those worst afflicted with fibromyalgia. Much of the information therefore is very negative, and for a newcomer with fibromyalgia it can all be a bit intimidating and indeed depressing.

Many people with clinical depression have some pre-existing personality traits and maybe even a family history of depression.

Fibromyalgia people have none of these.

Suicide is, unfortunately, one of the major problems in depression but is very rare in people with fibromyalgia. This is a rather dramatic statistical illustration of the difference between fibromyalgia and depression.

These assertions apply to the vast majority of people with FM, and are presented here to illustrate the view of the author that FM cannot be attributed to depression.

Some people with FM have been shown to be depressed, through suitably modified questionnaires, and it is important that any element of significant depression be recognised and treated appropriately in the same manner as might be an associated arthritis or systemic lupus erythematosis (SLE).

These points further strengthen the advice that proper medical assessment is necessary before you embark on any line of treatment, including that advocated here.

Overall while the majority of people with fibromyalgia might look depressed, and may even act as a depressed person might be expected to, the vast majority are not anything other than miserable as a consequence of their illness and its associated confusions.

Hypochondriasis

Preoccupation with health is not a feature of people with fibromyalgia. Indeed, the infinite majority of people with fibromyalgia would have been very irregular attendees at their doctor's clinic before they developed fibromyalgia. By nature, they tend to be people who declare that they were never a 'day sick' prior to their developing fibromyalgia or one of its associated disorders such as irritable bowel syndrome.

Once the syndrome develops some with FM become what can be termed body watchers. They tend to mentally scan their bodies for symptoms and attribute great significance to them all. However, this is a feature that appeared only since they developed FM. Therefore the suggestion that FM is a manifestation of hypochondriasis is invalid.

Viral cause

In earlier years, especially in people where fatigue was a prominent feature, it was felt that a virus triggered the disorder and that symptoms persisted because of a lingering viral infection.

Many viruses were implicated and some studies seemed to back up such theories.

These studies did not stand up to critical review, and there are very few who now accept that an ongoing viral infection can give rise to the chronic symptoms that are the hallmarks of fibromyalgia, even though it is known that a viral infection can cause increased sensitivity to pain in the short term.

Unfortunately, there are people with FM who wish to believe that they are victims of a viral infection. They feel that this will validate their claims of great suffering. It is very sad that they feel that they have to make efforts to validate the extent of their suffering. While it is understandable, it is regrettable, as it indicates that they do not understand FM. Unless they understand what they are confronting they will make no progress and will remain 'diseased patients'.

Muscle disorder

Even though it is absolutely accepted that sufferers have no inflammation in muscles, it has been suggested that muscle energy use may be abnormal, and that while the muscles look normal, they do not operate normally or use energy properly.

It has been suggested that this in turn leads to the accumulation of abnormal waste products which cause pain and fatigue. No studies have properly backed up these suggestions.

Microscopic examination of muscle fibres from patients when compared with muscle fibres of healthy people has revealed some abnormalities that were initially thought to be significant. However, when the muscle fibres of fibromyalgia people were compared with those of people who were not physically fit they were found to be exactly the same.

This really confirmed one of few points that are broadly accepted by most experts on the subject, namely that the vast majority of people with fibromyalgia are aerobically unfit. This perhaps is but another way of saying that they do not use provided energy optimally but it certainly does not suggest that there is any primary muscular disorder of any description.

Immunological disorder

No evidence has been found to suggest that any disorder of the immune system may play a role in causing fibromyalgia. However, just as in any chronically exhausted patient, there may be some minor immunological abnormalities that are of very doubtful significance. Most likely they are secondary to the presence of fibromyalgia and not at all a cause. In this respect they are similar to the hormonal changes.

There are many pseudo-scientific clinics with a vested interest in making people with fibromyalgia believe they have a disorder of the immune system who will take issue with this point. They are profitable clinics. Nevertheless you are going to succeed in regaining full health and a life of excellent quality without their help or even in spite of their help.

Social attitudes

Social attitudes to many disorders vary from time to time and from country to country.

This is especially the case in disorders that are poorly understood, e.g. fibromyalgia.

In Britain, for instance, there is much polemic discussion about Chronic Fatigue Syndrome (CFS) in both the medical and popular press where unfortunately the popular press and indeed many medical practitioners still refer to it as M.E.

Some claim it is a physical disorder, a silent epidemic caused by a virus, while others claim it to be a nonsense. There is much sentiment from both sides but no informed opinion and of course no facts. As earlier stated, media coverage of the topic has served only to entrench views already held by members of the population at large, based on how well sentiment on one or other side is presented.

In most countries fibromyalgia is accepted as a disorder, though many disagree about its cause or the effect it has on people. In the United States even those sympathetic towards the entity are aware of the fact that some people are jumping on the FM bandwagon for personal gain, which at the end of the day will diminish whatever public sympathy there is for people with fibromyalgia. It will also undermine the work of the many excellent scientists and doctors who are researching the subject.

Leading experts in the United States are also aware of what they describe as the beginning of the backlash against fibromyalgia. This backlash, already alluded to, concerns the concerted efforts of vested interests to ensure that you are regarded as some class of failure and that your suffering is not at all real. Basically, it will be a sad day for the many genuine victims of fibromyalgia if the significance of the condition is diminished; they will find themselves marginalised as in the past.

A positive social attitude can be rendered negative if the claims and aims of support groups are unreasonable, if opportunists use fibromyalgia for personal gain or if major financial institutions throw their financial might behind efforts to discredit it.

Medical attitudes

As earlier indicated many doctors find fibromyalgia very frustrating. That is fine if they admit as much.

There was an old medical adage that advised if a patient with arthritis came in the front door, the doctor's best line of action was to retreat out the back door! As treatment of arthritis has improved a lot this line of advice is now often tendered in the case of FM.

However, some practitioners without the backing of any knowledge, seek to lessen the significance of the disorder and the suffering of the victims. Many regard it as a psychological disorder and as such they betray at once a lack of understanding of fibromyalgia and/or a bias against psychological disorders as being real sources of suffering for many people.

Indeed many who accept fibromyalgia as a genuine entity make a similar error when they endeavour to rubbish the fact that psychological factors play a role in the suffering of fibromyalgia. Psychological factors play a role in the human ability to cope with any disorder.

Others, researchers in particular, see it as a complex disease of many systems of the body and feel that only medical science can crack it. They do accept that medical treatments thus far have proved useless, but believe that this should lead to them making even greater efforts to cure people with FM. In the meantime their attitude seems to be that you should wait for them to provide you with the answers to your problems.

Others believe that, with what is available they, individually, can taper the treatments to make their patients well or at least much better. This may be of some help but it still remains a fact that all treatments give poor results in spite of the positive attitudes of those genuine and enthusiastic doctors. However, this attitude at most can aspire to making your life with FM more tolerable while the aim of this book is to help you procure a life without FM.

Treatments Available

Treatments vary from the apparently logical to the utterly absurd. This book seeks to inform and educate you about FM so that you can help yourself. However, a brief reference to available and commonly-used, if quite ineffective treatments, is appropriate here.

Analgesics

Analgesics are painkillers and are often referred to as simple analgesics, to distinguish them from narcotic or more complex painkillers. Examples of simple analgesics are paracetamol (acetaminophen), low dose aspirin or low dose Ibuprofen.

More complex analgesics may contain codeine or dextro-propoxyphene and may have some pain modifying effects in the central nervous system. A small number of badly afflicted people may derive benefit from these or stronger medications of the same type known as narcotics. Having said this it remains the aim of the book to lead virtually all people to a totally drug free life and absolutely every one to a life of infinitely less medicine consumption.

Simple analgesics are by and large relatively free of side effects. Some people with fibromyalgia find them of some benefit but the majority of people do not derive satisfactory relief from them. Then again, this is par for the course, in fibromyalgia.

Anti-inflammatory drugs

Anti-inflammatory drugs are commonly called non-steroidal anti-inflammatory drugs (known by the acronym NSAIDs) or simply as non-steroidals. There is a multiplicity of these on the market. All have painkilling effects just as do simple analgesics and have some pain relieving value. They also have an anti-inflammatory effect in that they suppress inflammation, a quality that is much appreciated by many arthritis sufferers. They have many side effects especially in the gastro-intestinal tract and are not nearly so safe as ordinary analgesics.

As inflammation has nothing to do with fibromyalgia, many authorities are quite adamant that NSAIDs have no role whatsoever to play in the treatment of people with fibromyalgia.

However, many people with FM are desperate and some find them of some benefit, though logically they should provide very little help.

Muscle relaxants

Some medications allegedly relax muscles. Such medications are often based on the mistaken premise that increased muscle tension or muscle spasm plays a role in the pain of fibromyalgia. There is no evidence at all for such a suggestion. These medications can have at most a placebo effect, though Cyclobenzaprine which is a form of muscle relaxant is useful in improving sleep in some people with FM.

Tranquillisers

Because anxiety is allegedly apparent in people with fibromyalgia, many actually believe that it is a basic cause. This is not so. Tranquillisers are prescribed to alleviate the associated anxiety. In some cases there may be some, very transient, benefit. They are without basis for long-term treatment.

Anti-depressants

A number of anti-depressant medications are used, the most common of which is Tryptizol though many newer ones are coming to the fore, including Prozac.

Over the last number of years they have been used in very low doses to treat fibromyalgia. By very low doses is meant doses that are very small relative to the amounts that are used to treat depression. The logic of these drugs in these doses is that they allegedly increase the levels of substances, such as serotonin, that favourably influence pain control and sleep patterns. While they do have a logical basis, the bottom line is that they have not been proved to be of any significant benefit for any protracted period of time. This should serve to emphasise the fact that even medications that apparently have a logical benefit on the basis of present day understanding of chemical aberrations of FM are of very little practical use which in turn should strengthen your resolve to beat FM by your own methods.

This author rarely uses them and unless the person claims dramatic benefit, they are discontinued after six weeks. Their use for pain is not confined to FM. They are used for many chronically painful conditions where they seem to be of more use than they are in FM. As already stated people who may have major depression must be recognised and appropriately treated.

If such depressed patients do require anti-depressants they require amounts much greater than those used for the pain and poor sleep quality of fibromyalgia.

Sedatives

Sedatives are simply sleeping tablets. Many fibromyalgia sufferers believe they do not sleep enough. While their sleep may be a little more broken than that of people without fibromyalgia, this factor is not significant.

However, many people with fibromyalgia avail of sleeping tablets. They can be of some short term benefit but only insofar as they make the night less miserable. As the sleep deficit is one of sleep quality and not quantity, it would be a mistake for anyone with fibromyalgia to think fatigue will be alleviated by such medications in the long term.

Local injections

Multiple tender points are a feature of fibromyalgia. A traditional method of treating such tender points is to inject them with local anaesthetic or a combination of local anaesthetic and steroid preparation.

There are many reasons put forward to rationalise this line of treatment, but in practice the results are poor. Most doctors who have used them have given up on them after some years.

Physical therapy

There are so many treatments in this category that it is difficult to comment on them all.

Massage which is essentially a form of application of heat is of transient benefit to many, but whether it is superior to lying in a bath of hot water is debatable. Most people report vigorous massage as doing no more than adding to their pain.

Formal gymnasium-based programmes are not helpful. Perhaps the main reason for this is that the inevitably unfit person with FM will by nature push too hard and retire exhausted and demoralised.

Spinal manipulations or readjustments are utterly illogical, though advocated with tremendous zeal. The majority of people with fibromyalgia will only have their pain aggravated by such manipulative treatments.

Nerve stimulators

Trans-cutaneous electrical nerve stimulation (TENS) machines are widely used in many painful conditions. Whether they are issued in the belief that they are of any use, as a last throw of the dice, or something to keep the patient happy, is difficult to determine.

Most of them are technically very neat, and that perhaps is the best that can be said of them. By and large they are a bad prognostic indicator. Just as people who believe that a virus is the cause of their illness have a difficult road ahead, so also does anyone who will use one of these machines.

Indeed, if I see a patient arrive at a clinic with instruments of this type I know that progress is going to be most difficult.

Rest

Where fatigue is a very significant feature of fibromyalgia, rest has been advocated as a treatment. It has been suggested as the cornerstone of management and people have been advised particular rest programmes with the further advice that if anything hurts or makes you tired, then you should avoid that activity.

This usually means lying in bed all day or for as long as whatever takes the fancy of the multitude of advisors and health handlers that seem to have such ready uncritical access to the media.

No so long ago the advice was rest, rest, and more rest. I do not think anyone advises this method now. The one thing that studies have persistently revealed about people with fibromyalgia, is that they are aerobically unfit. In fact some of the earlier studies on the muscles of patients with fibromyalgia revealed abnormalities, similar to the muscles of unfit people.

Generally speaking people with fibromyalgia and more especially those labelled CFS are advised that they should do nothing to aggravate their pain and go to bed when they feel tired. Rest as a cornerstone of treatment is utterly illogical. If an unfit person walks three miles, for instance, he will be sore for the next couple of days.

No reasonable person would advise against such activity on that basis. Why then should different rules apply to equally unfit people with FM?

Fortunately, people of the fibromyalgia personality makeup find it very difficult indeed to lie about doing nothing physically or mentally, and they react very badly both physically and mentally to protracted periods of this ill-advised therapeutic measure. Rest has no role to play and is in fact detrimental.

Treatment downside

Treatments for all disorders have side-effects. There is no such thing as a medicine without side effects. Painkillers and more especially NSAIDs can cause stomach, liver, and kidney problems.

Sedatives and tranquillisers can cause drowsiness and problems with memory and concentration and sometimes dependency.

However, if you adopt the lines of management being advocated in this book then side effects will not be an issue as eventually medications will hopefully not be part of the equation.

There is another aspect of the medical treatment of fibromyalgia that is not widely appreciated.

Many people throughout the world have a degree of pain in their lower backs, perhaps from an incompetent disc. This large population of back-pain-victims can be broken down into two disparate groups.

The first group visit doctors or any of a wide variety of therapists and are avid consumers of whatever these therapists have to offer. In other words, they are patients and are dependent on physical, chemical or psychological products for well-being. The other group just get on with life. At most, they use a lumbar roll on a long car journey, avoid sitting for too long, and perhaps take a walk or a swim when the back aches excessively.

The first group are back-pain-patients whilst the second are people with back pain. The first group are dependants, the second group are people in control albeit with a nuisance of a disorder.

Consider the reaction to an increase in pain levels of the two groups. The first run for help. The second just do what they have to. This may involve avoiding gardening for a while, avoiding long periods of sitting, going for a walk, a swim, a sauna, a massage, or using a lumbar roll while driving. The former is a patient; a dependant. The second seeks to be in control and is in fact in control.

The same applies to fibromyalgia. You can choose to be a dependant-patient or a person afflicted by fibromyalgia. If you choose the former you are going nowhere.

This book obviously advocates the latter though it will take some time to liberate yourself from the shackles of the dependant-patient as virtually all with FM are medical patients in the long term and cannot understand how they could be otherwise.

The other downside of being a patient is that you abdicate responsibility for your own well-being to someone else even if you may regard them as successful professionals. That, they may well be, but you don't need them, their jargon, or their treatments in your efforts to beat fibromyalgia.

If you are of the patient mentality, you believe that it is your duty to passively accept whatever treatments are on offer. You are in effect waiting for an external solution. In other words, you are quite happy to remain a patient apart from occasionally complaining about how little progress is being made on your behalf by medical science.

You are giving responsibility for your well-being to a variety of people, and at the same time suppressing your inherent ability to recognise the condition for what it is, and much more significantly your ability to cope with it initially and to eventually overcome it completely.

The other major problem with modern medicine is that it informs you that all symptoms are evidence of a disease process and that you must have medical treatment to eradicate them. The same falsity is also propagated by the host of modern-day health-handlers and gurus of the alternative variety so prominently promoted by the media.

Part Two

Revitalisation

Introduction

The first part of this book tells you what FM is all about and why you may have been susceptible to its development in the first place. It also serves as a reminder to you that there is an understanding of your suffering. It must be viewed positively and as a firm base from which you will make progress to normal health and vitality. It will serve no function if you use it as a vindication for remaining a patient or to engender self-pity. Rather it should make you feel optimistic that you will enjoy a normal quality of life, even better than what you experienced before being affected by FM.

Part one also serves the purpose of educating those who care for you and helping them see the overall picture; those close to you will be very useful allies on the road ahead. At this stage, through your reading and reflection, your mind may be more open to new ideas and many of the myths you may have accepted as sacrosanct will have been debunked.

You should now feel optimistic as you have read some material that very many with FM have reported could have been written about them personally. Perhaps you also feel this way. In fact it is very much hoped that you do.

You should be further encouraged by the author's assertions that many people have completely overcome FM using the methods advocated here.

You are now ready to make progress in conquering this illness.

If you can embrace the mood and tone of what is written so far and if you can empathise with it, then it is time to positively address the important part of actually getting better, which is what it is all about. As the circumstances of no two individuals with FM are exactly the same there can be no absolutely specific recommendations but rather general guidelines that you should adopt, and adapt to your specific situation.

What you have to do is deal with the practicalities of fibromyalgia and use your knowledge to plot out your route to recovery. Standing on the sidelines observing academic researchers argue amongst themselves as to what is best for you should by now be alien to you. You should have rejected any notion that you are a long-term medical patient and that you should play no more than a passive role in your recovery.

Certainly, it is useful to be informed about developments in the academic field of fibromyalgia but you are aware that it takes years for research in various diseases to eventually benefit patients, and so academic research will not translate into immediate useful benefit for you.

By now, you must not regard yourself as a dependent diseased patient and while still suffering you should be ready to get on with it.

First Steps

It is widely accepted that current treatments of fibromyalgia are unsatisfactory and that many people continue to have symptoms for years.

Part of the reason for the failure of treatments is that they are used in a manner that suggests that people with fibromyalgia are physically or mentally diseased. The premise on which the alleged usefulness of this book is founded is that people with fibromyalgia, though ill, have no such physical or mental infirmity. Unless of course that you wish to regard the personality prototype that predisposes one to FM as evidence of a medical disorder.

Here it is contended that all of the symptoms and indeed the breakdown in the normal sleep and pain modulation systems, are secondary to over-burden in a personality type that takes on too much.

Research findings, relating to, for example, hormonal changes which affect stress coping mechanisms, are in no way incompatible with this fact.

As stated earlier, fibromyalgia is not due to stress, though this does play a role in the overall picture. As fibromyalgia is not a disease in the accepted sense, efforts at treating it as such are doomed to failure. It is for this reason that the rather florid term 'Revitalisation' has been chosen to describe Part Two rather than something like, 'Modern day management', 'Current treatments', 'Present day and future treatment strategies' or indeed 'Rehabilitation'.

All of these terms imply that you are a patient with a disease, rather than a person with a disorder. They also imply that your getting better is someone else's responsibility rather than your own, and furthermore that somehow you do not have the ability to overcome it without their assistance. They imply that, as best, you can be helped to cope better with an illness with which you must live.

This book challenges all of these assertions and seeks to put you in control of a situation that you can understand, contend with and eventually overcome, using your own natural resolve and resources. It insists that you have the inherent ability to beat fibromyalgia.

Coming to terms

Coming to terms with the disorder you have can be quite difficult even if you have not had any pre-conceived ideas as to its actual cause or effects, or indeed people's attitudes to it. It will be even more difficult for those with fixed ideas that they have a disease that must be cured, especially if they are receiving treatment from any of the proliferation of modern-day health-gurus or even from misguided medical practitioners.

However, there is no point in having recriminations about treatments that you have availed of and that did not work. Many have availed of these to some satisfaction. You also may have availed of them but if you are now trying the self-recovery route, then clearly you are not yet better.

There is not much point in looking back to the description of the symptoms of fibromyalgia in Part One of this book, and using it to convince yourself and others of your great suffering. Self-pity has no positive role to play and pity from others can quickly turn to annoyance and rejection.

It will be difficult to come to terms with the fact that your dreadful pain and fatigue is not due to some disease, but rather to a disorder that you will have to overcome by yourself.

This will be still more difficult in a society where the suffering of fibromyalgia victims is belittled by various vested interests. However, for you, nothing else has worked and you are now on this new and most likely the best, if not the only road, to recovery.

Accepting the diagnosis

Many people who are initially diagnosed as having fibromyalgia have trouble accepting the diagnosis; they may have the impression that they have been suffering from arthritis, or from some other more understandable disease entity.

They will also have trouble accepting the causes and nature of their disorder. This is a very great problem. In practice I find that those who can accept the diagnosis, its causes, and the recommended road to recovery, have a good chance of getting better, while those who cannot accept it or who do so reluctantly, will make no progress at all and will resort to the never-ending trail they were previously on.

There is little to be gained from going the route suggested here just because it differs from all others you were on and because it is unlikely to do you any harm. Neither should it be regarded as the last throw of the dice. It is not suggested that you should take it up with the zeal with which you previously adopted other strategies, but it is hoped that you will see alot of merit in it and embrace it with some enthusiasm.

Consolidation

It will take some time to take on board all that you have read, especially if you have been otherwise conditioned. This is a time for review and reflection. You may well have to read Part One of this book again in order to fully understand it.

In many cases there will be a certain amount of confusion and turmoil associated with this stage as it turns upside-down many of your understandings of the nature of the disorder and the proper way ahead for you.

You will also have to bear in mind that it is your own responsibility to get better. You will need to steel yourself in this resolve especially in the face of information that might suggest that much or all of what is written here is nonsense and that it is impossible to help yourself. This is a very difficult and courageous step to take.

You will have to embrace the self-help road rather than waiting for the medical cure that will never arrive. This involves avoiding various treatments that you might have recently heard of and not as yet have tried out.

Part of this process of consolidation is the task of enlightening your friends as to what fibromyalgia is all about, so that they can help you along the way. They will form an excellent alliance with you, to tackle a most formidable foe.

It will also involve assessing the way you lead your life and determining what factors rendered you susceptible to FM in the first place, what factors are still making a contribution, and more importantly how you can change them for your benefit. The road ahead will not be easy. Fibromyalgia must not be underestimated and the mere resolve to get better is not a guarantee of success any more than might be a resolve to lose weight, for instance.

Moving ahead

Even with everything going well, and with the support of friends, the road ahead is tough and long. It is far from easy sailing. In many cases, one step forward is often followed by two backwards. Just because you now understand fibromyalgia, does not guarantee that you have the strength to beat it.

This is especially the case if you have been suffering for a long time. For those who have not had the condition for a long time, it is possible to bounce back to normal health fairly quickly. The road is longer for those who have been demoralised and debilitated by a protracted period of life with fibromyalgia.

Part of the process that has led you to being so demoralised may have been the many frustrating encounters you have had with other methods of treatment.

You may also have encountered attitudes that have been cynical. And of course much of what is written about the subject is very negative and offers little hope. Indeed it has tended to advocate that you should sit back and wait for the medical world to make a major breakthrough. All this makes you passive and depressed. You have to shake off those negative forces before you can proceed.

However, no matter how far down you are you can still make it; it is possible to recover completely.

The first steps involve tackling what will be regarded as the more superficial aspects of fibromyalgia. These involve a determination to become well; acquiring physical fitness; renewing old friendships; developing pain-relieving and fatigue-relieving strategies.

The final more difficult and even more important steps involve tackling the fundamental substantive issues. This involves altering deeply ingrained attitudes that rendered you susceptible to the development of fibromyalgia in the first instance.

The significance of the difference between what I have referred to as the superficial and the core or more substantive issues cannot be over-emphasised. In your conflict, strength of resolve is but one of the essential ingredients in the amazing cocktail that will get you back to normal. Tactfulness and intelligence as well as your new-found knowledge are but some of the others.

Physical Fitness

It has already been mentioned that people with FM are aerobically unfit. Muscle biopsies indicate that the muscles are in poor condition. These problems can be rectified and that is now your most immediate responsibility and the one that you can most readily tackle.

It does appear that a good degree of physical fitness and conditioning protects against the pain of fibromyalgia, a point mirrored by many people's own experience.

Physical fitness raises your pain threshold and while it may not eliminate pain altogether, it does reduce its intensity and renders it less of a demoralising impediment in day-to-day living. This is not to say that the pain of fibromyalgia is due to lack of physical fitness, but that it can be greatly lessened by getting into good physical shape.

To advocate this line flies in the face of the advice that physical rest is beneficial in any way to sufferers of fibromyalgia. People with fibromyalgia know that increasing physical activity will aggravate their pain, and this is usually interpreted as a worsening of their 'disease' and therefore something that must be avoided.

This is a misconception which, in my view, hinders progress and one that should be totally discarded.

If a very unfit person jogs an un-accustomed five miles, she will be sore over the following few days. Is there anyone out there, who, on this basis will say to an unfit person that she is harming herself and advise her to refrain from such dangerous activity in the future?

Why then do different rules apply to the unfitness of a person with fibromyalgia?

Too much time has been spent and is being spent listening to medical advisors. One of the failings of modern medicine is its all-pervasiveness. Virtually everyone has a medically supervised birth, and death. All aspects of life in between are also medicalised. People today are instructed in what they should eat, what they should weigh, how they should engage in or enjoy social activity. Virtually everyone is a consumer of medicines, to the extent that it seems to be the role of one half of the people of the western world to be considered ill, and that of the other half to be doctors, therapists, advisors, counsellors, or health handlers of one type or another.

Even the healthiest of people today are patients. Olympic medal winners and top-class professional boxers have doctors, psychologists, therapists, nutritionists, and motivators of various types. A fit soccer player cannot resume play after being tripped without the application of some nonsensical spray, by a track-suited professional.

People are conditioned to believe that all physical discomforts are evidence of disease and must be eradicated by appropriate medical intervention.

The modern perception of the role of medicine has failed people with FM. Having got this far it is apparent that you no longer wish to regard yourself as anyone's patient nor indeed to regard yourself as a patient at all. Being a sufferer of FM means that you are almost certainly physically unfit and steps must be taken to rectify this.

In the experience of those with fibromyalgia, walking is the best method to achieve fitness. It is far superior to gym work which is supervised by a fitness trainer.

People with fibromyalgia are triers by nature and will want to keep up with everyone else, seeing virtually everything in a competitive manner, and for this reason formal gym work is undesirable.

Exercise programmes at home are tedious and do not help to get you out of the all too familiar confines of your home. Walking, on the other hand, can be done at your own pace and gets you out into the open air which in its own way is also therapeutic.

Walking is something you are fully in control of rather than a mere participant in what someone else, somewhere else, has designed. Already you probably have had an excess of what others feel is best for you. Walking is relaxing. It also involves expenditure of physical energy, and can help foster normal physical healthy tiredness as opposed to the dreadful washed-out exhausted way you usually feel. Perhaps it may also help invite a more natural sleep.

With regard to your walking programme, you should start with a reasonable distance that you can cope with. You build up the distance on a gradual basis. You must avoid the situation whereby you increase the effort on a day you feel good and then find yourself unable to go out next day. This is a rock on which many perish. It is pleasantly described by some people as the yo-yo effect.

If possible, bring a friend along with you. This will ease the tedium and lessen your focus on any discomfort.

At the end of some months your fitness levels will improve and your pain levels become less. The emphasis here is on improvement over some months rather than over some weeks. It is hard work but so very vital to your becoming well. At the end of this you will feel some sense of fulfilment at having achieved something by your own efforts.

The positive effect of this sense of fulfilment and of regaining control cannot be overestimated.

Renewing Friendships

People with fibromyalgia can become irritable and withdrawn. The first aspect drives friends away, the second leads to them walking away. Part of the revitalisation and your reintroduction to normal life, is to renew contact with lost acquaintances and friends.

It is vital to break out of your isolation to become the person you once were. These friends will not make the first move. It is up to you. This is not easy because whatever self-esteem you previously held will have been seriously dented by your illness and by the attitude of the many health handlers you may have encountered.

You will talk to your friends now in positive mode and hopefully with enthusiasm about the future as opposed to the negativism that up to now prevailed and that drove them away in the first place.

FM affects more than just you. Your family will have been involved, either by your malaise and unhappiness, or more indirectly, by their feelings of inadequacy in trying to help you. The help of family members will be required and if it can be procured it will be a tremendous asset.

Hopefully your new-found enthusiasm will lift some of the gloom that has also enveloped them and a feeling of optimism will prevail all round which will be further encouragement for you on your difficult journey.

Newly regained friends and family will now find you much easier to deal with and will enjoy meeting you again rather than regard such encounters as the painful experience they once were. You will find that your loved ones will respond in a much more positive manner than you might have anticipated.

Pain-relieving Strategies

The alleviation, if not the entire eradication of pain, while not in any way being the sum total of your ambition, is a very necessary part of your programme.

The treatments available for the pain of fibromyalgia are unsatisfactory so you will have to use what is available very judiciously rather than according to the protocols applied to disease states. You will have to be in control of all 'treatments', rather than accepting them and using them in a manner that is appropriate to other disorders. These strategies do not work for you and must not be blindly and helplessly availed of.

Many people report that heat, whether it be acquired by a hot shower, lying in a bath of hot water, or massage, is an effective if temporary reliever of the pain and stiffness of fibromyalgia.

These should be availed of as you see fit.

The same should apply to your use of painkillers (analgesics). While you may find them of little use, others do derive some benefit from them.

If you derive significant benefit from a painkiller, then you can avail of it as you see fit. Do not take it if it does not give a certain amount of relief. You do not take it on the basis that your pain is so bad that it appears natural and necessary to take something.

You must manage your pain and your painkillers. Do not allow painkillers to manage or control you. Use them wisely and judiciously at your discretion and at your discretion only. Use them for your benefit. Only you can decide on how to maximise whatever good they do for you, bearing in mind that they are but temporary supports on your road to being a medication-free zone. The ultimate achievement of normal health will bring with it the need for no painkillers or any other medications for FM.

Basically your attitude to your painkillers changes dramatically. If you need them you use them; you control them, not the other way about. Do not grasp at them in helpless desperation as might a drowning man grasp a straw.

You are now beginning to take charge. Fibromyalgia sufferers are often very enthusiastic about liberating themselves from medication. Being a patient does not come naturally, or rest easily with them.

Quite apart from the poor efficacy of medication, the fibromyalgia population as a whole is inordinately sensitive to the side effects of medications.

The main reason why most people with fibromyalgia stop taking medication is not because they are not deriving any benefit from it, but because it is causing side effects.

This is a further example of how your attitude to medication has been wrong. You are likely to have stopped it because it was harming you, and not because it was doing no good.

You were instinctively using medicine. Now, in either case, with your new perspective you stop medication in the first instance if it is doing no real good, and you also stop it if it upsets you.

The same principles must be applied to medications such as Tryptizol or related drugs. These low dose anti-depressants however have a slow onset of action and you either use them on a regular basis, or not at all.

Unless you feel they are doing an enormous amount of good, then they should really be the first tablets to go, if only for the fact that you cannot control them like you can painkillers. Likewise anti-inflammatories should be eliminated if at all possible. As stated, a small number of patients do derive benefit from some narcotic drugs but even if you are in this category this book will hopefully help you.

A certain number of people with FM will also have depression, for which treatment is required. You do not attempt to alter or discontinue drugs or other treatments used for depression without the advice of your medical practitioner, no matter how enthusiastic you may be to get off drugs.

This does not apply to low dose Trytizol to nearly the same extent, and which in your case may only be for the pain and fatigue but you should still consult you doctor if you wish to come off it.

In a nutshell, with regard to pain, you now control what you consume rather than being a pathetic hapless consumer of what you are being fed by others, taking medication only because you don't know of anything better.

All medications have a placebo effect. On this basis if you discontinue pain-alleviating medications you may temporally feel a bit more pain. Do not be discouraged by this.

A transient period of a little more pain should be easy enough to bear, as a little more pain makes very little difference when you are in severe pain all the time. Your improving levels of physical fitness will more than compensate for this and your improving morale will render it relatively easy to handle for the short period it will last.

Besides it is a very positive step you are taking a major step forward, and this should also strengthen your resolve to see it through.

Pain management clinics

This is the type of self-help book that seeks to put you in control of your own destiny. Its aim is to help you initially to understand FM and eventually overcome it. Its intention is not to help you manage the pain or other symptoms of FM, but rather to beat it in its entirety.

Fibromyalgia cannot be managed. If present, at all, it is in control. It has to be beaten and its many heads cut off one by one.

A visit to a pain management clinic is an option. If you elect to avail of it, you check it out and see what it has to offer you. It may suit some and not others. As with most other aids in fibromyalgia a pain management clinic is just another aid.

It will not rid you of fibromyalgia. Your aim is not to learn to live with fibromyalgia, but to learn to live without it. You do not hand yourself over to a clinic to be cured. It cannot be done. Only you can take all the steps that count.

In reality, it makes no sense to deliver yourself to a clinic and expect them to cure you. This is the way many people mistakenly approach pain clinics. You, on the other hand, armed with your new-found knowledge, if you choose to visit one, look around and avail of whatever parts of it you feel might fit into your overall plan. By now you should be formulating an overall strategy.

With regard to the pain clinic you should imagine you are in an exciting outlet store, but on a limited budget. In such a case you buy what you need essentially, rather than what you might like.

If you go to a pain clinic take from it not what the sales persons offer, but only what suits you. You then use that to help yourself to become well rather than expect the clinic to make you well on its terms.

Tender point injections

These are relatively harmless, and not of much benefit overall. Again you may avail of them sparingly if you find them of benefit. They are not a long-term solution by any means. If you find them helpful, good and well. Only your assessment again is valid.

Analgesic sprays

These are of many types and have little to recommend them scientifically though in the main they are harmless and you may find some of them of temporary benefit. It seems like alot of choices are being left to yourself, but no-body said it would be easy.

Fatigue-relieving Strategies

The most fundamental part of contending with the fatigue is to avoid extreme inactivity which can only worsen the situation. Just as walking serves to raise the pain threshold, it will improve also physical fitness and will help alleviate the fatigue that is often associated with inactivity.

Many of you will appreciate that teenagers who spend their time watching television or playing computer games generally complain of having little energy.

Sleeping tablets get you to sleep and keep you in sleep for a longer period but they do not improve sleep quality. If used on a constant basis their consumption should be reduced and they should only be used on an irregular basis. If you have trouble getting off to sleep they are reasonable for short periods but other strategies more conducive to quality sleep should be used.

The more relaxed you are the better the choices are of quality sleep. To suggest replacing coffee with hot chocolate would be a patronising slight of your intelligence.

Whatever you find relaxing whether it be reading, listening to music, a walk or physical work out, yoga or massage should be availed of as you see fit while the sleep-enhancing aspects of enjoyable sexual activity are known since time immemorial.

Just as in acquiring physical fitness, and in alleviating pain, you will have to devise your own methods to procure good quality sleep and you will have to appreciate the severe limitations of all types of medication.

Progress

At any rate you must now be getting the picture. Medication, doctors, therapists, may be invited by you to be part of your team. But you are the captain in control, subservient to, and dependent on no one. This status you must attain before commencing on the rest of your journey which is even more difficult, as it tackles the core issues. The outlook is forward, positive, and optimistic.

It is hoped, at this stage, that friends and loved ones will also have moved into a position whereby they can help you to make progress. Invite them to read this text so that they know that the situation is not hopeless. Some progress can be made in a matter of weeks. However, it is generally not very substantial at first assessment. At perhaps 6-8 weeks, many who endorse what is written here, report that the pain levels are just a little improved. Many, do, however, report that their exercise tolerance has improved and that they are able to walk greater distances.

Some are disappointed at the slow rate of progress but many report that they are optimistic about the future for the first time ever. They also generally have cut down quite considerably on the amount of medication they are consuming and they are greatly encouraged by this as they would have felt in the past that these medicines or other treatments were critical to survival.

Survival is not what the game is all about but rather the acquisition of normality.

At this early stage they often report that they have not as yet reached out to renew friendships, but that they intend to. Even more encouraging is the fact that many say that they have read the information supplied here, and that it has given them a great insight into what it is that ails them and more importantly, an insight into the factors that have caused them to become unwell. The most encouraging statement that can be made, is that a person experiences a sense of gaining control.

Another satisfactory statement one frequently hears from the person with FM, is that family and loved ones have read the information provided, have identified with it, recognised the nature of the problem and expressed a desire to help. All does not go as well as this so quickly but even in the first couple of months some of these positive features at least have come to the fore.

At the very worst, virtually every person will state that even if they have not made much progress they are absolutely adamant that there is no way that they are going to allow themselves to deteriorate further. By this they mean that they have formed a steady firm base from which the only way to go, is up.

Hopefully, your experience will also be positive. If you have not already done so, it is now time to reach out to your former friends. Over the phone they will know by the tone of your voice that you are somehow different, somehow more like the old you they once were friendly with. Conversations with friends are now optimistic.

You engage in conversation. Your friends are not subject to a depressing monologue. They even suggest further meetings. Things are certainly looking up!

On the other hand there are a small number of people who may report that they have read what is written here and find that it offers no help at all. They will ask how, in this modern age, can so little be done to help. Even at this early stage, it is clear that these people are going to have a very difficult road ahead.

Some will also report that they tried walking and, almost accusingly, report that they are now worse. Clearly the route advocated here is going to be very difficult for them.

This may be due to the fact that they had too high a level of expectation from dealing only with the superficial issues or it may be due to the fact that they did not actually deal with them as well as they thought they had. They should not give up, as dealing with the core substantive issues described in the next chapters will provide more benefits. On the downside, however, is the fact that if one fails with the easier more superficial issues then she is less likely to be able for the last lap.

The Last Lap

If you have taken on board all that has been written so far, if you can see that it applies to you, if you have accomplished such tasks as regaining physical fitness, renewing acquaintances, making allies out of friends and family and if you do not now regard yourself as being diseased and in need of medical treatment, then you are ready to embark on the last and most difficult part of your marathon task.

Do not feel exasperated at the suggestion that it is even more difficult than what you have had to do before. If you have achieved the goals mentioned above, you are now a much stronger and more formidable person than you were before you tackled FM.

By now your confidence levels will be much higher than before and of course the sense of well-being you will have acquired from doing something for yourself and by yourself alone for perhaps the first time in your life, will have made you a much stronger person still.

All this new-found strength will be required in order that you should be able to complete your journey. Being better than what you were initially is no achievement in the overall context of your conflict. Only total victory will suffice. Either you or FM is in control. There is no compromise, no truce, no acceptable level of FM in your life.

You are now standing steady on your own two feet and who dares suggest you cannot complete the journey to success! Indeed, you may well appreciate that you have got further than ever you thought possible, so why limit yourself now?

The last step will be the most intriguing of all. Up to now you have learned alot about FM which is critical to ultimate success.

Now you are going to learn alot more about yourself. When you combine your knowledge of FM with your new deeper understanding of yourself you will be well prepared for the final lap. The relatively straight-forward route so far is to be replaced by a different set of strategies. You are now going to deal with the more substantive issues.

The last lap should be viewed with enthusiasm and excitement as its completion will ensure a quality of life for you that you could never have believed possible and one better than you enjoyed before fibromyalgia entered your life.

What you have achieved so far is to have dealt with the more salient aspects of fibromyalgia. You have learned much about the condition, you have resolved to overcome it, you have resolved not to be a patient and you have achieved some degree of aerobic physical fitness. You also have renewed friendships, re-acquired a social life, and hopefully incorporated loved ones into your plan. You are in positive rather than passive mode.

What now needs to be dealt with are the roots of the disorder that are deeply embedded in your being. This cannot be done unless you have the capacity to understand the complexities of your relationship with others in your world and, more significantly still, with yourself.

The most striking feature of the fibromyalgia population is the similarity of the personality prototype. It is clearly advocated in this book that this personality type uniquely predisposes all its bearers to the development of FM. While no one can suggest that there is anything wrong with this personality sub-set, and indeed it does bestow many great strengths, it has in truth played a very significant role in your developing FM.

Perhaps it might be more true to suggest that associated with this personality type are a large number of attitudes and perceptions that have led to your taking on so much, that in turn led to the upset of the sleep pattern and the pain control mechanisms and thus the symptoms of FM.

These attitudes need to be altered as they are the major contributory factor to your ill health. They are the substantive issues already alluded to.

There are many different aspects to these attitudes that for practical purposes can be roughly divided into three sub-groups, all of which are in need of radical change. What requires change is firstly, the attitude of others towards you, secondly your attitude towards others, and lastly your own attitude towards yourself.

The terms of reference of all relationships that are influenced by these attitudes must be assessed, re-appraised, and altered for the better. As some of these attitudes have been deeply ingrained most likely since your formative years, the task ahead obviously will be difficult. In some respects suggestions that you alter these attitudes is akin to asking a leopard to change his spots. The excitement at the prospect of such an intriguing challenge should give you an inner strength that you did not believe you had rather than leading you to accepting that it cannot be done.

Again only general guide-lines can be offered. They should be intelligently adopted and incorporated into your overall programme.

The Attitude of Others Towards You

By nature those susceptible to the development of FM are intense, meticulous, perfectionist type personalities. This leads them to do everything to the highest standards possible. They are very intolerant of anything not being done to their own high standards.

In the workplace they can be relied upon to do everything correctly. This is a good thing in itself but it can lead to others developing an attitude that is not helpful.

The more you do, often the more is expected of you. Likewise you are frequently expected to produce perfection even when the framework within the working environment is not up to acceptable standards. Far too often, it is assumed that regardless of circumstances you will produce the goods. Management can fall short in providing the necessary back-up. They know that you can compensate for these shortcomings by your own initiative and more unfortunately by your having to drive yourself to excess.

This, rest assured, is nothing personal but it is the nature of management to only look at the end results. If the end results are fine then there is no stimulus to provide a working environment that would ensure equal efficiency but with fewer demands being made on you. While you are around, fellow workers can do much less work or even slovenly work, as you will be unable to resist your urges to see that the end result is perfect.

This is a pitfall most people with FM fall into. After some time it becomes the 'modus operandi' of your work environment and you end up trapped in a situation, partly of your own making, whereby you are doing far too much work to compensate for those who are only too happy to sit back and let you do it. Indeed your fellow workers may feel that you are revelling in this role. For a while you may well have enjoyed this role, but a stage will arrive where this situation is damaging your health. If you have FM, that stage has already arrived. At the end of each day you are now drained. While your fellow workers can go home and relax with friends and family and indeed enjoy friends and family, you are so worn out that you are incapable of such enjoyment. The day has taken everything out of you and you have nothing left to give yourself or anyone else.

Your initial get up and go has got up and gone! The price you are paying for this excessive devotion to duty is not just that you are extremely tired at the end of the day, but you are also paying the price of missing out on family life.

While you are in part co-author of your own misfortune, it is equally true to say that the attitude of your co-workers towards you is the major contributory factor. Their attitude towards you needs altering.

This can only be achieved over a period of time. People with FM do not expect very much for themselves but when you consider that this is also having an effect on your relationship with friends and family and indeed the quality of life of friends and family, it should encourage you to get moving and ensure that something is done about it.

You will have to move tactfully along this road. You must remember that you will be seeking to change a situation that may have prevailed for many years. In some instances you will be stepping on some people's toes. To be fair, most of these people may not have realised that the attitudes they have acquired towards you were and remain a contributing factor to your ill-health. When this is made clear to them, in a tactful manner, many will be prepared to smarten up their own act, to ensure that you are not excessively burdened. People will generally be receptive if you deal with the situation in a discreet and non-confrontational manner.

With those who will not co-operate, you will need to be more firm.

It is probably true that you have never stood up for yourself and it will not come naturally to you to do so now. However, your efforts will be fortified by the knowledge that their attitudes are not alone harming you, but are also harming the life quality of your loved ones by virtue of their being denied access to your true and vital self. Therefore if it makes you feel any better you can assure yourself that you are taking these steps not just for you, but for your family and friends.

Of course, your own self-interest and well-being should be sufficient inspiration but that is another story.

If co-operation is not forthcoming you can always have recourse to the help of management. The vast majority of people with FM underestimate the esteem and value in which they are held by management and are very pleasantly surprised to find that managers are only too willing to ensure a better work environment for them. If that does not transpire to be the case and if help is not forthcoming due to a bad work environment or unenlightened management, then you must give serious consideration to getting out of it altogether.

It is absolutely imperative that you should try to change the attitude of others rather than backing out because you feel it cannot be done. It is better to fight the good fight and lose in the boxing ring, as it were, than to concede without trying. This may well be the first time you have ever stood up for yourself and, even if you do not get the desired result, the fact that you have made the effort will do wonders for your self-esteem and your ability to assert yourself, qualities which are in short supply in fibromyalgia sufferers.

If you are in management the change may be a little easier as the altering of attitudes may essentially involve delegation of duties. This is easier said than done as most with FM would prefer to do things themselves rather than having to look over the shoulders of others, not so dedicated, to ensure things are done properly.

Overall if you are in management and if you are not delegating properly, then you are not working in an efficient manner and you may well be surprised that when you effect all the changes that are necessary for your own health, productivity actually increases but at considerably less cost to you. The work environment will be happier and healthier for all concerned.

Perhaps for the first time in your life you are now experiencing a degree of control, experiencing what it is like to be actively doing things to your own agenda rather than reacting to the consequences of the attitudes of others towards you. You will likewise command much more respect, where people actually appreciate you for what you are rather than for what you can do for them.

Many people with FM experience this and will relate the fact that it does really feel good. There is no reason why this should not also apply to you, but you have to make it happen.

Again it needs to be stated that you cannot make any moves until you have appraised the situation thoroughly and intelligently.

You must ensure change with discretion and common sense. There is no point in accepting that the attitudes of others towards you are playing a role in your ill health, and approaching the matter like a bull in a china shop. There is no point in endeavouring to make people feel guilty about how they treated you and no point in seeking sympathy.

What you want is to effect change for the better, and you do not want to alienate those who will be of most assistance to you on your road to recovery.

Fortunately most people with FM are blessed with at least average intelligence and while they may have a tendency to be too forthright, their intelligence and more significantly the vital necessity of success should ensure that they move in a discreet and sensible manner. Deviousness and subterfuge serve no purpose but fortunately these are not traits possessed in abundance by those with FM.

People with FM have an inherent desire to feel needed and useful to others. For that reason many are involved in charitable and voluntary organisations. Here also they give too much of themselves and if you find yourself in this position you should endeavour to give less of yourself and not to over-burden yourself still more.

In such charitable organisations you may find yourself in a position that exactly mirrors the one in the work place. Obviously, getting out of such a situation is easier than dealing with a similar situation at work.

Altering the attitudes of others towards you in the work-place will be difficult but if the problem lies in the area of personal relationships, it is even more difficult to deal with.

Women of the FM personality prototype are often the strong force in most relationships, especially in marriages with children. Women in most cases are responsible for the rearing of the children and play the role of confidante and confessor for them. Females with FM often carry too much of the psychological burden of all relationships they are involved in. Indeed, many a relationship is founded on the premise that the female will carry such emotional and psychological burdens. Thus, while clearly unfair, it often is a major contributory factor to the development of FM in any person. Perhaps this is one of the reasons why the condition is so much more common in females.

If this is the case, the attitude of the one not carrying an equal share of the burden must be altered. This can be very difficult in some cases. In others it may not be so difficult. Many such people are not to be blamed for the attitudes society ingrained in them and many partners when they realise that their attitude is a problem have successfully transformed themselves, much to the surprise of the person with FM.

If you are fortunate enough to have such a partner then you will do very well, as there is no doubt that the help of loved ones is the single greatest asset you will have on the journey to normal health.

Some people with FM make the mistake of using the information acquired here to lay blame at the feet of the one who inadvertently contributed to their being over-burdened. This may be an effort to gain pity or to make the other person feel guilty. It is a negative attitude. You do not want to punish anyone. Sympathy is the last thing you need. Sympathy and pity are short-term attitudes that can quickly turn to contempt.

One-up-man-ship and scoring points in a relationship that in itself is going through an unhealthy phase, serves no useful purpose.

It is an attitude unworthy of anyone with FM and one that will almost certainly ensure failure in the long run.

There are, however, situations where a partner will make no effort. If that is the case, then that person values the comforts of the current situation more than he does your well-being and more than he does a more normal, satisfactory, mature relationship with you. If this is indeed the case it is best to cut your losses and get out before you are so broken up that you will never be able to put the pieces of your life together again. Obviously, there are situations in which addictions, substance abuse, infidelity or aberrant social behaviour precludes any change in the attitude of the partner. You should be able to recognise an irretrievable situation quickly, salvage what you can, and get out.

It is true, but very unfortunate, that many women in these situations blame themselves. It is even more unfortunate that supposed professional medical helpers also see them as the problem.

This may be especially true in fibromyalgia. For people with FM much professional help is directed at the innocent victim as though she were the problem. Much of this mindless professional activity is directed at patching her up and fortifying her into further accepting and enduring a situation that is causing her such ill health. Indeed, it is just as well that medical treatment for fibromyalgia is as bad as it is. If it were better, all it would succeed in doing is to maintain an unsatisfactory and unhealthy situation that would never be intelligently appraised.

Overall you must survey the situation and if it is possible to change attitudes towards you, then you should have the courage and skill to go along that road. If it is not, then you should have the wisdom to recognise the situation and the courage in these cases to get out without any feeling of failure or self-recrimination.

However, in the vast majority of cases it is possible to alter the attitudes of others and many people with fibromyalgia succeed in doing so by their own efforts once they are sufficiently educated in what they are confronting.

Your Attitude Towards Others

This obviously is linked closely to the attitude of others towards you. The basic problem with the attitude of people with FM is that they feel they should ever please and be pleasing to others. Up to a point, this is an admirable trait, a little of which is needed in all members of a civilised society. Such selfless devotion may be useful to missionaries but in day-to-day living when excessively expressed and unconditionally tendered, it does not work out for the good and is a health-hazard. It really cannot be healthy to measure your worth only in terms of your value to others.

However, many with FM are most comfortable when giving to, and doing for, others. This has helped shape unhealthy attitudes towards you. Many people enter relationships with others on the basis that they should be ever pleasing. This attitude leads to the development of an immature and unsatisfactory relationship.

Like the quality of mercy a mature and healthy relationship involves the graciousness of giving and receiving in somewhat equal measures. If either or both partners are forever giving or taking, the relationship can never be healthy but will always be strained even if those involved in it cannot see it because they are too close to the wood in order to see the trees.

Just as it is the attitude of others to expect too much of you, it is your attitude to be always giving and expecting nothing in return. Therefore, your own attitude is contributing to the problem and it needs altering. This can be quite difficult as many people, even those without FM, have difficulty in receiving and are at ease only when giving. It can be suggested that it is as selfish to wish to give all the time, as it is to receive all the time. It can be further suggested that it is more difficult to alter the first personality trait, that of the permanent giver.

At first sight there may not appear to be much to be gained from the changing of your attitude towards others. However, it must be clear that it directly influences the attitude of others towards you and it should be equally clear that it is at once both impossible and futile to change one without changing the other.

If you are forever giving then you are inviting more than your share of burden. Physical burdens you most likely can cope with. However, in personal relationships you may invite upon your shoulders excess psychological and emotional burden. This most people cannot carry and if you have FM you certainly cannot carry it.

You are not a professional counsellor or psychologist or an expert in relationships. Unlike the professionals, you cannot turn off and unwind at the end of the day because no day has an end for you.

You are therefore obliged for your own well-being to alter the attitudes you hold that helped lead to the development of the problem. This is imperative if you want to overcome FM. If successful, you will have the added bonus of a fruitful, mature, and satisfying relationship with both friends and loved ones. They, also, will benefit from the more sensible parameters of the new relationship and may well express satisfaction with this.

Attitudes Towards Self

People with FM define their worth only in terms of their value to others and they expect very little for themselves in return. Life is to be endured, not enjoyed. They are uncomfortable with leisure time. When they should be relaxing at home and enjoying time out with the children, for instance, they are frequently to be found buzzing around cleaning and re-cleaning, tidying and re-tidying. This busy little housewife role has been idealised in old western films and should be thus confined.

In the business world of today it is now being realised that you are more productive when not totally stressed out. The same applies to life generally and will be shown to be so when someone takes time out to think.

Take time out to reflect on your attitude towards yourself. You should start by ensuring that you have some leisure time each day regardless of the demands of others. While you will initially feel guilty about this and while you will find it hard to handle, you need to train yourself to overcome these self-imposed obstacles.

Different strategies can be used. Meeting a friend for coffee, a walk, or a jog will get you away from the immediate environment in which you find so much to do, whether it needs doing or not.

If friends or loved ones are causing psychological over-burden then they need to be tactfully guided towards assuming more responsibility for themselves. If there is little prospect of them doing this you have to realise that your well-being is your top priority and the relationship may have to be terminated.

You have to treat yourself as well or at least nearly as well as you treat others. You must be easier on yourself and more forgiving to yourself as you no doubt are to others. Do for yourself what you would gladly do for others.

This new attitude towards yourself involves putting your own interest and well-being up there with the interests and well-being of others.

This is not advocating selfishness, but rather maturity in relationships. It is suggesting that you should be a normal, complex, functioning human being.

A peculiar feature of all of this is that you are endeavouring to change your very defining features and traits as others see you. It is your distinguishing characteristics of absolute reliability and being there selflessly for others that needs altering. Given that these hallmarks have likely been present since childhood, you can appreciate that it is not going to be easy and that you need a lot of confidence and wisdom to achieve it.

Of course after taking reasonable care of yourself in day-to-day living, if you have anything left in excess you can dispense with it as you see fit.

Up to now you were expending all your physical and mental energy on other people's needs, and using what, if any, was left for yourself. The new situation turns this old way of doing things on its head. You look after yourself primarily and give what's left to others. This is not selfishness; it is practical action. If you are unhealthy you are of less use to others than you would wish. These others at any rate should want you for what you are, and not for what service you can provide them with.

At the end of the day all attitudes including those of others to you, of you to others, and finally of you to yourself, need appraisal and change.

A satisfactory conclusion must be reached. There are no half measures. There can be no compromise with FM. Unless eradicated completely it is in control. All of this changing of attitudes is obviously much more complex and much more difficult to achieve than are the earlier steps of relaxing and acquiring physical fitness.

However, very many people do achieve just this and their reward is being at peace with themselves and with their environment. This allows the restoration of the normal sleep pattern and pain control mechanisms, the disruption of which are the primary physiological flaws that give rise to the symptoms of FM.

Changing of attitudes is a difficult task and it may appear that very little is being offered here to take you to success. You cannot be brought to success. You have to grind out each step of the way, by yourself. But rest assured that each successful step gives you a boost that helps you take the next one.

All that can be offered in this book is education and knowledge of the nature of FM, as well as some general guidelines on the road to recovery. The circumstances and the energy levels of people with fibromyalgia are never the same, so there can be no such thing as a step-by-step guide to success.

Step-by-step guidelines are only for people who are intellectually lazy. This fortunately is an uncommon trait in the FM population. A high input of intellectual energy is required in overcoming fibromyalgia, hence the provision here of only general guidelines.

In a similar vein you can see now that to rely on medicines or health-gurus to make things happen for you is a lazy option that will get you nowhere.

Can Anyone Help?

Progress in FM is often slow and frustrating. Your conflict is certainly very difficult and very different to anything you will have undertaken before. Even if you accept all that is written here and endeavour to move along the lines suggested, you may feel you are getting nowhere. This is especially the case for those people who make some progress only then to have setbacks before they can consolidate what gains they have made. Likewise, it is only human nature to feel, in spite of what has been explained to you, that this book does not do enough for you. Please rest assured that the idea it contains have helped many people to recover from what were very devastating states.

You may feel that the book insists that you do everything on your own, except for the help of friends. You may feel that it belittles professional help in a patronising manner. It does not seek to do this but it does point out the futility of some well-meaning treatments and makes you aware that there are many bad treatments available also.

While it does clearly indicate that all useful steps have to be taken by yourself it does not in any way rule out availing of some professional help. The emphasis here is on availing of professional help and on using professional help, not subjecting yourself to professional help. Far too many people, with far too many problems, hand themselves and their well-being over to professionals and, for a fee, expect to be made better.

This serves no purpose, especially in FM. It simply cannot do so because of the nature of the disorder and its many complexities.

If you wish to avail of the help of professionals you must do so on your own terms, not on theirs. You choose what suits you. If you feel tense and uptight or unable to relax then there is no reason why you cannot use yoga, aromatherapy, or meditation. You assess its usefulness, having tried it. You determine if it helps you or not.

You do not hand yourself over to a therapist and say 'Make me better; that is what you are being paid for'. You do not allow them to assess your progress or indeed to make any suggestions as to how you are doing. Only you can determine how you are progressing. You must be in control regardless of whether the therapist is comfortable with that or not. If the therapist has a problem with you not being a passive recipient of what he or she has to offer, then you must go elsewhere.

Your attend these treatments to ensure progress and to get results. You do not go just to fool yourself into believing that you are doing something. Occasionally people with FM will say, 'I have done this and done that as recommended but I am no better and what are you going to do now?' They will say that they are now walking X miles per day and that they have given up some charity work or that they have employed a cleaner to lessen the amount of work they are doing, or have attended some relaxation classes and yet are no better.

Many such people have missed the point of this book. They have addressed and dealt with many of the more superficial aspects such as achieving physical fittness and off-loading excess physical burden. But they have not as yet dealt with the major substantive issues such as the changing of attitudes and rendering relationships more mature; changes that are fundamental to progress. They also may have failed to incorporate friends and partners into their programmes.

In relation to treatments and using professional helpers, the important point is that you should avail of treatments on your terms, to achieve something concrete. You do not avail of them just because it seems to be better than doing nothing. Obviously you do not avail of such dreadful spurious therapies such as having your spine or sacro-iliac joint realigned. You do not go to countless sessions of physical therapy to have treatments directed at areas of alleged muscle spasm and tension.

What you must do is escape from the dependent-patient role, avoid being molly-coddled by various therapists, and take charge of your own destiny. You avail only of treatments you find useful, rather than treatments that others tell you are useful.

You should avail of the help of friends. This is essential. Clearly you will have driven away a number of friends during your periods of negativism. Now you speak to them with optimism and ask them to help you make progress rather than ask them to listen to your meanderings as you may well have done in the past. Friends will rally very quickly especially when they detect new positive notes rather than the old negative tone.

You may well wish to know why it is that you are so demanding of self why you expect so little of others and possibly why your self-esteem may be low. Again the advice of any intelligent psychologist, counsellor or friend may be availed of. You must not allow these people to take you over or treat you as a patient or a psychological-inadequate who needs patching up. These people should only be employed to help you clarify the overall picture but not to sort it out for you. Only you can effect any necessary changes.

You do not need them to make a diagnosis, as you have one already. They may be able to offer some general guidelines. You do not follow any instructions blindly. You assess any advice they give you for what it is, and incorporate it into your programme for self-revitalisation. You do not allow yourself to be incorporated into any programme of their liking.

If you feel that they are wresting control from you, then get out and go elsewhere.

You will determine whether such people are of help to you by assessing their intelligence and willingness and enthusiasm to help you. You will not be impressed by jargon or specific formulas; the latter are often the hallmarks of well degreed but non-intelligent technocrats. These people and their services are to be used to help you get better on your terms and are not to be used as psychological crutches to help you keep going as you are. They are to be used to help you to effect the changes necessary for your well being. You avail of the services of professionals only as long as you feel they are helpful. Their assessment as to whether you are making progress or not is of no great interest to you. Only your assessment is valid. You are not their patient. Indeed, you are nobody's patient. You are a customer. If their product is of use to you then purchase it sparingly, and use it as you see fit.

If problems lie in relationships and you and your partner want to but cannot on your own improve matters, then a relationship counsellor may be of benefit if he/she is on your wavelength. The idea is to elevate the relationship to a higher plane, not to patch up a doomed relationship.

At this stage you should have the overall picture. These counsellors or psychologists must be on your wave-length and not the other way about. Many of these people assess you as a school teacher assesses a child. You are a good child if you blindly accept their dictates and a bad rebellious child if you do not.

Counsellors may present you with some unpalatable facts that you would rather not hear about. If so, you can be pretty certain they are trying to help you rather than have you tagging along while being told what you want to hear. The last thing you need is some sort of comfortable symbiotic relationship which will result in nothing being achieved. This scenario is all too common.

Overall, all sets of relationships between you and others and between you and yourself, must be re-appraised in a cool and calculated manner and where they are based on wrong sets of values and are damaging to your well-being, they must be altered.

It has to be glaringly clear at this stage that medications cannot possibly be of any help when you reach that stage of your revitalisation process that involves the altering of all of the attitudes that have been written about.

Further Progress

As conquering fibromyalgia involves so much, progress can be slow. Given the amount of misery it causes it could never be expected to be otherwise. Some people with FM are further down than others and the duration of their recovery can be expected to be longer as they do not have adequate levels of physical or mental energy to initiate the process straight away.

They also find it much more difficult to bounce back when the inevitable temporary setbacks occur.

Some people do not receive the required help and so their course is very difficult. Some live in horrible circumstances and escaping from FM can be all but impossible. Some do not have the intelligence to understand what it is that ails them and so make no progress. Some may still insist that they have a disease rather than a disorder and it is the duty of others to fix them. Such people remain as they are. The majority of this group get worse and become more embittered with time.

Obviously nothing changes for those who, for secondary gain, assume the symptoms of FM, but such people are not the concern of this book any more than is anyone with genuine FM who has accommodated to it and desires only pity, rather than a life of normality.

To make progress you need to accept what is written here or else your commitment will be lukewarm. Beating fibromyalgia requires utter conviction and one hundred per cent commitment. This you cannot give if you have doubts about the course of action you are taking. Only you can tell if you are doing well. In medical journals, believe it or not, authors of published articles consider that a reduction in pain levels and a reduction in the tender point count, represents improvement. This is fine for those assessors and indeed they can compare notes with other doctors but it has no practical application to you.

You know how you feel and you should feel insulted if anyone were to tell you that your tender point count is improved. This pseudo-science, even if it achieves that dubious status, has no bearing on your conflict with fibromyalgia.

It is a crazy method of assessing any individual with FM, as fibromyalgia is a situation where you, and only you, are the one who can assess progress.

Progress will continue relatively slowly. This is to be expected as it does take time to implement all the changes necessary for the recovery of health. With walking, stamina and fitness improve in some months and with it pain levels. The other features do lag behind but the majority of people with the right attitude and hopefully appropriate help from those about them make significant progress in 6-12 months.

You must however realise that there can be set-backs on the road to recovery and you must not become demoralised or have your strength or will to succeed by your own efforts curbed in any way.

Success will be yours at the end of the day. Many people when they beat FM report they now enjoy a quality of life superior to that enjoyed before fibromyalgia became a part of their lives. There are a number of reasons why this might be so.

In the first instance there is the sense of achievement at having overcome a most formidable disorder. It is also true that people usually have a higher appreciation of their health and vitality after a period of illness. This latter point cannot be over-stated.

You will have learned much about yourself on your journey. This new-found knowledge of yourself can in many ways help you to better enjoy the rest of your life and indeed improve the life quality of those you care for.

Likewise people about you will now see you in a different light, further improving your sense of self-worth. Your relationships with people will be on new terms and you will not feel the need to be forever pleasing. In essence all relationships will be more mature and thus all the more fulfilling.

Finally you will have the added sense of achievement when you realise that perhaps this was the first time ever that you took control of your life, that you acted positively in relation to your own requirements, rather than forever reacting to the needs of others and to your need to please. Self-esteem will have been established.

It is a very exciting prospect and one that is eminently attainable with intelligence, education, and hard work, no matter how far down you may be, with fibromyalgia.

Life After Fibromyalgia

Life after fibromyalgia in a sense resembles life after the liberation of body and soul from some terrible sentence. The real you has been reborn and you have learned a new way to fly. Your low level of expectation of life of any quality has dissipated. Life is now being enjoyed rather than being endured. The addiction of always having to please others has been overcome. You do not have to prove yourself anymore.

You are more relaxed with yourself and with your environment which is why the normal sleep pattern and pain control mechanisms have been re-established.

Your home life has improved. Perhaps each pane of glass and each tile on the floor is not as spotless as it was in the past, but this is more than compensated for by the new air of tranquillity and peace that permeates the place instead of the tension that once reigned.

Friends now are looking forward to meeting you and that feeling is mutual. The quality of life of loved ones in your immediate personal environment also improves just as yours does.

You now do your work with a healthy diligence rather than with an unhealthy passion for ultra-perfection. This does not equate with becoming slovenly but rather indicates that you have liberated yourself from the impossible aspiration of doing all things better than anyone else.

It is maturity. As tension eases all around, and as the maturity of all relationships improves, so does life quality for all.

The pains, fatigue and the need for medications and other treatments have also gone. Pain and fatigue are the symptoms of an underlying disorder, just as is a temperature often a manifestation of an underlying infection. Bringing down the temperature does not eradicate the infection. In the same way easing the pain or fatigue if that were possible, would do nothing to improve the underlying disorder that gives rise to them. Indeed, it was the undue pre-occupation of victims and medical carers with the pain, tender point count, and fatigue, that prevented progress being made. No one ever really looked past them to determine the real nature of the problem in fibromyalgia and chronic fatigue syndrome.

You now know better and that is why you have succeeded regardless of the opinions of others.

You can now move on with your life.